D0088331

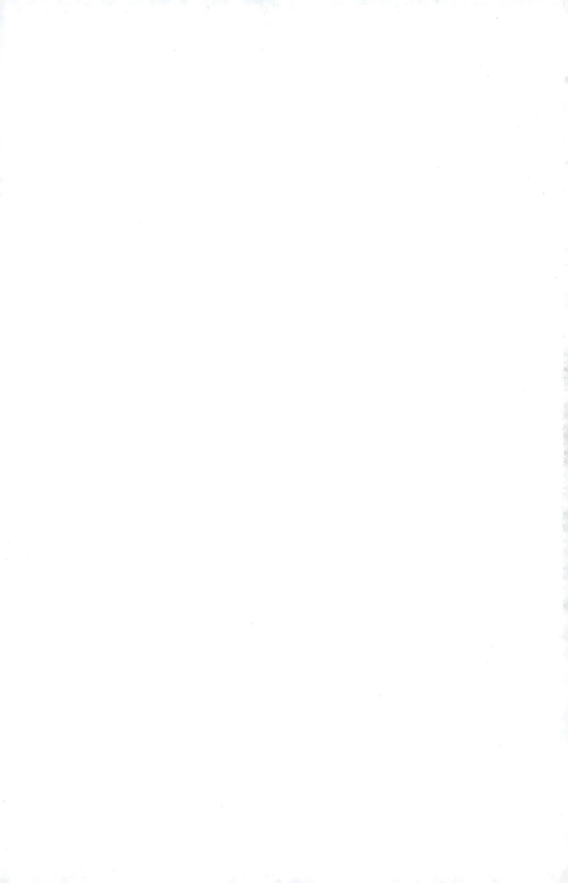

REPRODUCTIVE RIGHTS AND THE STATE

**Recent Titles in
Reproductive Rights and Policy**

REPRODUCTIVE RIGHTS AND THE STATE

Getting the Birth Control, RU-486, and Morning-After Pills and the Gardasil Vaccine to the U.S. Market

Melissa Haussman

Reproductive Rights and Policy
Judith A. Baer, Series Editor

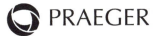 PRAEGER

AN IMPRINT OF ABC-CLIO, LLC
Santa Barbara, California • Denver, Colorado • Oxford, England

Library of Congress Cataloging-in-Publication Data

Haussman, Melissa, 1959–
    Reproductive rights and the state : getting the birth control, RU-486, and morning-after pills and the Gardasil vaccine to the U.S. market / Melissa Haussman.
        p. cm. — (Reproductive rights and policy)
    Includes bibliographical references and index.
    ISBN 978-0-313-39822-3 (hbk. : alk. paper) — ISBN 978-0-313-39823-0 (ebook)   1. Reproductive rights—United States.   2. Birth control—Government policy—United States.   3. Birth control—Law and legislation—United States.   4. Contraceptives—United States.   5. Women's rights—United States.   I. Title.
    HQ766.5.U5H387   2013
    363.9'60973—dc23   2012027447

ISBN: 978-0-313-39822-3
EISBN: 978-0-313-39823-0

17   16   15   14   13   2   3   4   5

This book is also available on the World Wide Web as an eBook.
Visit www.abc-clio.com for details.

Praeger
An Imprint of ABC-CLIO, LLC

ABC-CLIO, LLC
130 Cremona Drive, P.O. Box 1911
Santa Barbara, California 93116-1911

This book is printed on acid-free paper (∞)

Manufactured in the United States of America

*. . .it is so important that being a woman is
not a preexisting condition as a part of
our health care system.*
*—California Congresswoman
Lynne Woolsey, March 18, 2010*

Contents

Series Foreword

These are bad times for women's sexual and reproductive freedom. Restrictions on abortion have made that choice more difficult, while *Roe v. Wade* remains one Supreme Court vote short of extinction. The precarious status of abortion rights is old news. Until 2012, however, women's right to prevent pregnancy seemed to be noncontroversial. That state of affairs abruptly changed. I did not expect ever again to hear a sexually active single woman called a slut—then Rush Limbaugh did, on his radio show. The segments of the population that have insisted on abstinence-only sex education for teens now expect adults to remain celibate outside of marriage. The Roman Catholic Church, whose handling of its child-abuse scandal has destroyed whatever moral authority it possessed, is suing for an exemption to the requirement that employers include contraception in their employees' health insurance. Although 17 percent of the members of Congress are women, birth-control policy is set there by an exclusively male group. A large and vocal segment of American society seeks to deprive women of the freedom to act and to control the consequences of their acts.

Emergency contraception, Plan B, or the morning-after pill offers women a unique opportunity to deal with the consequences of heterosexual intercourse after the fact, not before. The procedure is not quite birth control, but not quite abortion either. Melissa Haussman's study brings a comparativist's perspective to what was once a peculiarly American phenomenon: the transformation of reproductive health from a medical specialty to a political controversy. (The fact that, in the spring of 2012, the prime minister of Turkey is calling for the recriminalization of abortion suggests that this phenomenon is no longer American.) This book lucidly situates Plan B within the ongoing struggle over reproductive choice. The long, difficult struggle to make emergency contraception available led Haussman to the insight that "women's reproductive rights have never been front and center of the U.S. policymaking framework. Instead, they are treated for their mobilizing potential, usually for external constituencies."

This political process did not start with Plan B, and it seems unlikely to end there. Eugenicists who wanted to stop the unfit from procreating were as active in the early birth-control movement as feminists were. (In fact, some early feminists opposed birth control because they thought it made women more vulnerable to their husbands' sexual demands.) The record of the birth-control pill provides a telling comparison with the fate of Plan B. If we look only at outcomes, the histories appear to be polar opposites. The pill was rushed onto the market in the 1960s, inadequately tested, over the misgivings of the Food and Drug Administrations. But Haussman's analysis of these two episodes in pharmaceutical history shows that the processes were similar in their ranking of political and economic concerns over women's health issues.

The pill had the enthusiastic support of the major pharmaceutical companies and such diverse groups as the Planned Parenthood Federation of America, the American College of Obstetrics and Gynecology, and the Playboy Foundation. There was no feminist movement to take a position. The primary opponent was the Roman Catholic Church, which lost the battle. Who won? Certainly, Big Pharma did. So did the ob-gyns who were rewarded for endorsing and prescribing the pill. The FDA, unable to warn doctors and patients about possible side effects, suffered a setback. Men—at least, the sort who read *Playboy*—gained from the transfer to women of the responsibility to prevent pregnancy. Ultimately, women won, once the estrogen dose was lowered and the side effects decreased. But the first cohort of women who took the pill became guinea pigs for this experiment.

By the time Plan B was ready for use, the feminist movement was a major player in American politics. Feminists perceived emergency contraception as increasing women's control over their lives without the risks accompanying the first oral contraceptives. Big Pharma had the same economic interests that had motivated the companies with DES, the pill, and hormone replacement therapy. Their inability to promote their interests as smoothly as they had in the past had nothing to do with women's political power, but was the product of significant changes in political climate and religious demographics since the 1960s. The resurgent conservatism that has influenced and sometimes dominated American politics since the Reagan administration has emphasized family values, which take a dim view of sexual freedom outside of monogamous heterosexual dyads. The Christian right may be neither, as the joke goes, but evangelical Protestant groups have joined with the Roman Catholic Church in reaction against the sexual revolution and its instrumentalities. This book gives little ground for optimism and much for pessimism.

Judith A. Baer
Series Editor

Acknowledgments

First, I must acknowledge the fact that Professor Judith Baer, series editor, political science professor at Texas A&M University, provided me the inspiration to write this book when she asked me to do so at an annual meeting of the American Political Science Association (APSA). As sister members of the APSA Women's Caucus and Women and Politics Research Section, we have been familiar with each other's work for years and often have sat on panels together, describing, discussing, and postulating about the status of constitutional law in the United States and other countries and roads to improvement.

The book that I consider a direct predecessor to this one is *Abortion Politics in North America* (Lynne Rienner, 2005). Judy and I thought this would be an interesting next step in my research into the ways in which the U.S., Canadian, and Mexican political systems have all worked more often than not to thwart access to women's reproductive rights. Occasionally, there are windows of opportunity that get opened to savvy and tenacious women activists, but normally a long period of work and strategizing precedes any such opening.

As always, I dedicate this work to my patient spouse Linda, and to my network of family and friends. Specifically, I want to honor the lives and work of the North American-based network of dedicated pro-choice workers and providers.

1

Introduction

This book was written with the understanding that women's ability to control their lives rests fundamentally with power over their reproductive choices. This discussion shows that the desire to enhance women's power has not been central to U.S. reproductive drug policymaking. While pharmaceutical companies, federal and state governments, and pharmacies could help women, they have at times abdicated that responsibility based on stated fear of pro-life pressure. More often, the purported pro-life pressure is a cover for government and pharma's fear of damage to the bottom line of the for-profit U.S. pharma sector. Despite the fact that women are the majority of the U.S. population and consumers, they do not have any level of policy power proportionately resembling their strength in numbers. This study is also a clear call to elect more responsible, pro-choice women to office at all levels and to encourage them to become pharmacy owners and key players in pharma companies. In this way, women will have the decision-making power to help women control their reproductive decisions. In this scenario, the women in the public and private-sector offices would be effecting both descriptive and substantive representation.

At the one point in time where public and private-sector decision-making coincided to favor women's interests, from the mid-1950s to 1973, the overall ethos was not to help women, per se. Rather, this period was one where the

U.S. pharmaceutical, agricultural, and chemical industries sought and received government and foundation-based funding, largely from Rockefeller and Ford, to develop and test their products. The testing usually took place off the official U.S. radar screen, in Latin America, Asia, or in the U.S. territory of Puerto Rico. When these products—including miracle seeds and rices and contraceptive injections, devices, and pills—were developed, they were then typically publicly subsidized. In that manner, all countries and all users in the United States could afford access to the technology.[1] Donald Critchlow has shown how John D. Rockefeller III, as head of the Rockefeller Foundation, worked to fund and develop contraceptives, including the birth-control pill developed by Dr. Gregory Pincus. Presidents Johnson and Nixon put public funding for contraception for low-income women in their budgets, to be administered through the Health, Education, and Welfare Department (which was split into separate Education and Health and Human Services Departments in 1979). Critchlow details how Rockefeller was able to broker a consensus with the U.S. Catholic Church not to lobby against public contraception funding for low-income women, while they retained the authority to preach against chemical contraception in their parishes.[2]

Critchlow also discusses how the 1973 *Roe v. Wade* decision irrevocably drove the Catholic Church out of the silent majority, allowing contraception to be publicly-funded and into the arms of the since more powerful pro-life (sometimes also called "pro-family" coalition). The pro-life and pro-family distinction is made by William Saletan, who describes Catholic groups' mobilizing since 1973 around the principle of never favoring anything that would harm life. On the other hand, fundamentalist Protestant groups' membership in the coalition is sometimes based on a slightly different principle, that of promoting marriage but also limited childbearing.[3]

Another blow to hopes of pro-choice strength after 1973 was the downfall of both the liberal bloc, including the Rockefellers (particularly after the death of former Vice President Nelson Rockefeller), and the pro-contraception/pro-choice consensus within the Republican Party. Part of this shift was demographically based, with the rise of Sunbelt politics following Nixon's Solid South strategy, as formulated and chronicled by Kevin Phillips.[4] Under Nixon, the Republican Party began to switch its appeal to Southern white conservatives, largely fundamentalist Protestants. To this coalition were added Catholics in huge numbers, the Reagan Democrats of the 1980s. As termed by Nixon, the "Southern strategy" provided an opening for the conservative, pro-life, and pro-family strands into the inner circle of the Republican Party and certainly into the inner circle of reproductive policymaking. The newly powerful bloc included Senators Jeremiah Denton (R-AL) and Orrin Hatch (R-UT) in the Senate and Representatives Don Nickels (R-OK), J.C. Watts (R-OK), and Robert Dornan (R-CA). Also aiding this effort was the rise of well-funded and well-organized conservative lobby groups, including Americans United for Life (AUL), the National Right to Life Committee (NRLC), the American Life League(ALL), Focus on the Family (FOF), and the Family Research Council (FRC). These groups were dedicated to reversing the *Roe* decision and blocking Planned Parenthood's pro-choice work in the United States, and managed to pass many different measures concerning how and where abortions are performed and cutting out low-income funding for abortion and contraception.

In many ways, the groups that had worked hard to normalize contraception provision as part of a national framework in the United States through the early 1970s and had worked on abortion law reform were blindsided by the quick emergence of the pro-life and pro-family groups (largely called pro-life in this book as a shorthand). Groups such as Planned Parenthood Federation of America (PPFA), the National Abortion Rights Action League (NARAL), the spin-off group Abortion Rights Mobilization (ARM), and the National Organization for Women (NOW) were all knocked on the defensive, and NOW was quite busy in the 1970s with the state-by-state ERA (Equal Rights Amendment) campaign, also something against which the pro-life community worked.

Alarmed by the string of pro-life successes after 1973, the pro-choice movement worked in the 1970s to try to stall the legislative and judicial impediments thrown up to abortion, contraceptive, and overall comprehensive sexual health services access. The 1989 *Webster* and 1992 *Casey* decisions, ironically both authored by libertarian Justice Sandra D. O'Connor, were the result of many test cases litigated through the states by the NRLC and AUL. These two cases legitimized many areas of state legislative power to restrict surgical abortion access; funding restrictions had already been put in place through the 1976 Hyde Amendment and the conscience clauses began with the 1974 Hatch Amendment. Most states copied the Hyde formula banning public funding for abortion, many extended that to contraception, and within a decade after *Casey* more than 500 abortion-restrictive laws had been passed at the state level.[5]

The response of the pro-choice movement was to try to expand women's options. The first strategy began in the mid-1980s in trying to gain U.S. access to the French formula for RU-486, the medical abortion pill, based on a combination of mifepristone and misoprostol. This effort was spearheaded and led throughout by Lawrence Lader, founder of the original NARAL (National Association to Repeal Abortion Laws) in the 1960s. He worked on the RU-486 effort as the head of his own organization, ARM, in concert with Eleanor Smeal, head of the Feminist Majority Foundation (FMF), and with Planned Parenthood. The efforts of ARM, the FMF, and Planned Parenthood were first to try to convince

Roussel-Uclaf, the patent holder, to push for U.S. approval. Roussel was reluctant to do so, claiming the threats of pro-life boycotts against its more profitable drugs. Fears for the bottom line similarly trumped any potential concern for women's rights when all other major U.S.-based pharmaceutical companies, having profited handsomely from investing in women's reproductive drugs since the 1960s, refused to patent RU-486 and work for Food and Drug Administration (FDA) approval.

Pro-choice advocacy groups, aided by the research-based U.S. Population Council, persisted by locating labs willing to manufacture copies of RU-486 (the Danco Lab in New York state). Lader found a Chinese manufacturer, the Hua Lian company, which had simply manufactured its own unlicensed version of RU-486 and provided it to millions of Chinese women. Under the Clinton administration, particularly Secretary of Health and Human Services (HHS) Donna Shalala, the Population Council acquired the patent from Roussel. The FDA announced its approval toward the end of the second Clinton administration, in September 2000.

The issue of emergency contraception has played out in a strange way in the United States. The first type of pill was a combination of synthetic estrogen (estradiol) and progesterone (levonorgestrel), given in higher than usual dosages and invented by Canadian doctor Albert Yuzpe in 1974. In the United States, it was licensed by the Gynetics Company, a maker of endometrial curettes. In 1998, the Preven kit, containing a pregnancy test package, information, and the pill combination, was approved by the FDA on a prescription basis. In 1997, the FDA stated that emergency contraception was a safe and effective way to prevent pregnancy after sex. The FDA based its conclusion on 10 studies conducted since 1977 using high dosages of combination hormonal pills.[6] The argument for emergency contraception is that there are roughly three million unintended pregnancies in the United States each year, about half of them are due to contraceptive failure and about half of them end in abortion. Used correctly, within 72 hours after sex, emergency contraception could prevent most unintended pregnancies.[7] The Yuzpe method had been studied in World Health Organization (WHO)-sponsored studies since the 1980s.[8]

The second half of the emergency contraception picture is found in Plan B, at first a two-pill progestin only combination of levonorgestrel, currently available in a one-pill format. Developed by Barr Laboratories in the 1990s, it received approval from the Reproductive Health Advisory Committee of the FDA in 1998. In 1998, the FDA Advisory Committee suggested that Plan B could be made over the counter (OTC) for distribution in pharmacies. In 1999, the FDA approved it on a prescription-only basis. While the Clinton administration's

HHS secretary, Donna Shalala, and FDA commissioner within the department, Jane Henney, were able to get RU-486 and both types of emergency contraception through the FDA on a prescription basis, the opportunity structure changed drastically with the inauguration of the George W. Bush administration in 2001 with former Wisconsin governor Tommy Thompson as HHS secretary and M. D. Mark McClellan, associate professor of health economics at Stanford University, to be the FDA commissioner.[9] McClellan came from a well-known Texas political family and his brother Scott was President Bush's first press secretary.

The WHO sponsored a large-scale study of the Preven versus Plan B pills starting in 1999. By the time the studies were in, conclusively demonstrating that Plan B was the better option, the Bush administration was in place. In 2003, Barr Labs followed up on the FDA's 1998 recommendation to submit an application for Plan B to be distributed OTC. In 2003, the FDA Advisory Committee issued a report supporting the move to OTC status for Plan B, by a vote of 23 to 4. The tide started to turn against Plan B in 2004, just when Preven had been taken off the market in anticipation of Plan B approval. In February 2004, a 90-day hold was placed on the FDA's decision, and by May 2004 the FDA rejected the switch to OTC stating that not enough data was in place for females under 16.[10] Ironically, two years later, the FDA considered the new drug application for Gardasil, and while there was a noted lack of data for women under 13, approval was granted in June 2006. At that time, a new HHS secretary (former Utah governor Michael Leavitt) was in place with a new (acting) commissioner of the FDA, Andrew von Eschenbach.

One part of the pro-choice advocacy coalition's strategy to move Plan B was contained in a report commissioned by Congressman Henry Waxman (D-CA) prepared by the Government Accountability Office. The 2005 report excoriated the FDA for ignoring its own Advisory Committee's advice and stalling FDA approval on the OTC question. Following this, the leadership of the FDA was subpoenaed for congressional testimony, and the secret testimony revealed conversations between the FDA head and staff in the Executive Office of the President to stall OTC approval. The second was a lawsuit brought against the FDA by the Center for Reproductive Law and Policy (CRLP; changed to the Center for Reproductive Rights [CRR] in 2003) for ignoring its own timeline between Advisory Committee approval and required FDA action. The CRR's second goal was to publicize the secret FDA testimony. As this suit was wending its way through Federal District Court in New York, the Bush administration suddenly dropped its objections and Plan B was given OTC status for women 18 years and older as of October 2006. It was only extended to 17 year olds after another CRLP lawsuit in March 2009, with the FDA decision made in April 2009. Despite these actions, there has been a record of inconsistency in pharmacy availability across the United States, due to the variety of pharmacy and insurance regulations at the state level.

In Chapters 5 and 6 on RU-486 and Plan B, respectively, the question of social movement organization learning is taken up, describing women's response after decades of dealing with the male-dominated private-sector pharma bureaucracy and public-sector legislative and executive branches. Savvy women entrepreneurs, including Beverly Winikoff, M.D., and Sharon Camp, Ph.D., either formed (Winikoff) or headed (Camp) small companies to provide the interface between pharma and the U.S. and other governments. Beverly Winikoff formed Gynuity in 2003 after a 25-year history as director of reproductive health at the Population Council. The company has been an important liaison to the offshore manufacturers of RU-486 and the WHO in getting it added to its formulary. Dr. Camp, after 18 years as senior vice president of Population Action International, became the president and CEO of the Women's Capital Corporation, formed in 1997 to shepherd Plan B through the FDA process. A different story is told in Chapter 7 about Gardasil, where the Merck Company co-opted preexisting women's groups to lobby for it. The three central groups that functioned in this manner were the Cancer Research and Prevention Foundation, the Step-Up Women's Network, and Women in Government. Some may have viewed the relationship as mutually beneficial, since Merck generously rewarded these groups when they increased awareness of or legislation on, first, cervical cancer and, second, Merck's monopolistic presence in the field (prior to 2009). Others, however, clearly saw Merck as using women, particularly state legislators and celebrities, to be the public women's faces of the multimillion dollar campaign.

LITERATURE REVIEW

This book's analysis draws from the new institutionalist framework, primarily because its central task is to explain how U.S. political and private-sector institutions have ignored women's reproductive drug needs since the 19th century.[11] Probably the best-known strand of institutionalism is historical institutionalism, which, as its name sounds, describes how political institutions developed in response to crucial events and constituencies. In the United States, historical institutionalism overlaps strongly with the American political development (APD) approach. The preeminent FDA scholar using this approach is Daniel Carpenter, whose book *Reputation and Power: Organizational Image and Pharmaceutical Regulation at the FDA* yields an understanding of how historical forces inside and outside of the agency led it to take certain policy choices.[12] Carpenter adapts the 1962 two faces of power framework of Bachrach and Baratz, where those controlling institutions could affect others through either decisions or non-decisions.[13] In applying the Bachrach and Baratz framework to the FDA, Carpenter expands it to three faces of power. In Carpenter's study, the first type of power "to make others do things" is called directive and the second one of nondecisions from Bachrach and Baratz becomes that of "gatekeeping" of the agenda and access to institutional power in Carpenter's theme. Carpenter adds a third type of power, conceptual, that forms a large part of his study in describing the FDA's actions to maintain its reputation as the world's pharma gatekeeper.[14] Carpenter's third type of power, conceptual/reputational, relates how FDA actors have worked to keep certain images of the agency in the public's mind.

Another compelling account in the general APD area is Stephen Ceccoli's *Pill Politics*, using Frank Baumgartner and Bryan Jones's "punctuated equilibrium" model.[15] Ceccoli's explanation is related to FDA change based on "focusing events." In the punctuated equilibrium model, focusing events are the only ones that can interrupt relatively long periods of institutional stability. In the Baumgartner and Jones model, focusing events are viewed as "exogenous shocks" to the institution in question. In this model adapted by Ceccoli, the typically closed "iron triangle" of influence between Congressional committees, the FDA, and pharma has been interrupted a few times to change the FDA in some crucial manner.[16]

The four subsets of institutionalist theory include historical, sociological or organizational, discursive, and rational choice institutionalisms. Historical institutionalism examines how institutions can be created and continued by political forces that then embed their views of how an institution should function in its future workings.[17] Historical institutionalists may see an institution as essentially path-dependent, whereby a specific policy becomes its central focus, blocking out alternatives, or in a different mode, called "constant cause" by Mazur and McBride.[18] The path-dependent model essentially specifies that the earliest ground rules are then set up as impediments to future change. However, the constant cause model, including punctuated equilibria, allows for change in institutions, typically wrought by outside forces. Both types of historical institutionalism are relevant for large and complex institutions such as the U.S. Congress and executive agencies. For example the male, heavily resourced overrepresentation within them has tended to continue since their creation, showing path dependency. However, it is also possible to apply the constant cause model to the U.S. political system at times, such as Ceccoli has done for the FDA. A congressional-presidential example would be the arrival of Presidents Kennedy and Johnson in office in the 1960s and their work to perform end runs around intransigent Southern conservatives to ensure passage of the 1964 Civil Rights Act.

In addition to the well-known historical models, two other types of institutionalist theory are sociological or organizational institutionalism and discursive institutionalism. There is seeming overlap across these two subcategories that can lead to confusion. Both are said to address institutional change from within the organization. Mazur and McBride, citing Vivien Schmidt, describe discursive institutionalism as being based on the role of ideas in the institution: "the way individuals and groups in the institutions develop and communicate ideas, and the patterns and effects of their discourse."[19] Mazur and McBride describe the discursive type as being about change in the institution from inside. However, Krook and Mackay assign a similar meaning to sociological/organizational institutionalism when they describe it as emphasizing frames of meaning guiding human behavior and the interactive character between institutions and the individuals in them.[20] Since both categories emphasize the role of ideas and the power to control the dialogue with them, they must be seen as complementary theories.

The final type of institutionalist theory described by Krook and Mackay is rational choice institutionalism, which tries to "understand the origins of institutions, the mechanisms of their survival and the nature of their effects on macro-political outcomes."[21] Since all of these criteria are also important to the path-dependent and constant cause subsets of historical institutionalism, it again is difficult to draw a wide dividing line across them. It is usually a matter of degree to differentiate the strands. From the point of view of the American political development school, all of the factors and strategies outlined in the four strands of institutionalist explanation are certainly relevant to explaining the historic tin ear of U.S. pharma and the FDA to women's concerns.

This book acknowledges the utility of theoretical strands that link events inside and outside institutions, for that is the key emphasis on how the FDA and other parts of the HHS department grew to be the creatures they are. In recognizing the strategies of framing of policy options and political campaigns, this analysis certainly engages in discursive and organizational or sociological institutionalisms. It also often describes actors, particularly pharma, as weighing cost-benefit analyses and thus employs a form of rational choice institutionalism.

There are two major stumbling blocks for any empirical study using institutionalist theory. The first is how exogenous versus endogenous influences are defined. Some of the literature, for example, defines exogenous forces as a different level of government, so that the federal U.S. government becomes an outside force affecting the states' policy options. That seems a drastic separation. In Ceccoli's model, to be discussed mainly in Chapter 2, exogenous shocks included the thalidomide disaster of the early 1960s. The degree of that event's characterization as an outside shock could be questioned since the FDA was heavily involved in it. Endogeneous influences are easier to cover, of course, since one can usually describe who is represented in an institution and who is not. The bottom line of this book is to examine both sets of influences. The inclusion of both yields the most realistic assessment of where U.S. pharma policymaking has been impervious to women's influence and where it has in certain cases been made to confront it.

The second, larger question for institutionalist scholars is how to decide change in policy or institutions is happening, and how to measure and explain it. Wolfgang Streeck and Kathleen Thelen provide a thorough overview of institutionalist theories in *Beyond Continuity: Institutional Change in Advanced Political Economies*.[22] Tracing the beginning of the current waves of comparative theory to Paul Pierson regarding the welfare state and Peter Hall to capitalism, they note that most accounts tend to emphasize continuity much more than change.[23] Regarding theories of change, they note a vast uncharted middle ground in institutionalist theory between path-dependency, emphasizing how only incremental changes can happen over time, and the large ruptures envisioned by punctuated equilibrium theory. Streeck and Thelen posit different types of gradualist institutional change that proves helpful for the discussion in this book. The first type of gradualist institutional change covered by Streeck and Thelen is displacement, often described in the organizational/sociological strand of institutionalism, whereby new models emerge to delegitimize previous organizational practices.[24] The second is called layering, argued by Pierson, in which previously embedded allegiances and structures in an institution form costly obstacles to change.[25] Streeck and Thelen view layering as possible when "institutional structures are highly change-resistant but the political environment is conducive to reform."[26]

The third process referred to by Streeck and Thelen is drift, whereby an institution or policy may appear stable on the surface, but does not respond to political shifts. Drift can occur when "neither internal structures nor political contexts favor reform."[27] Under a scenario of drift, the institution's reach into an outside constituency changes. The institution–constituency relationship changes because the institution has stopped adapting, thus some constituencies are no longer covered by the institution's policies. This model is strongly emphasized by leading U.S. social policy theorist Jacob Hacker. He describes changes to the U.S. pension and insurance system since the 1980s as reducing the coverage of the population's risks all while appearing to maintain the same ground rules established at the start.[28] Hacker's work is quite helpful to this book because he believes that putting the study of risk protection policies at the center of welfare state development yields a clearer picture of welfare state development than the usual studies concentrating on income redistribution.[29] Hacker's description of subtle shifts to the system of U.S. private insurance as off-loading risk coverage is of great relevance to the central concerns of this study. For example, it helps to describe the tug of war over Republican versus Democratic control of the U.S. Department of HHS and the FDA and the policy results.

The two other types of gradual yet profound institutional change discussed by Streeck and Thelen include conversion, in which institutions are redirected to new goals or functions.[30] Conversion is likely to occur when "institutions are highly-malleable yet substantial barriers block authoritative change," and the rules are changed from within.[31] It unhappily coexists with drift as an explanation for the anti-women policies of the FDA under President George W. Bush. The final type of change is called exhaustion, in which an institution basically collapses under its own contradictions.[32] One of the central ideas of historical institutionalism is that different agencies (or parts of an agency) may change at varying speeds. Some parts of a political institutional structure may thus be adapting to changed circumstances, while others do not. For the purposes of this analysis, the clearest policy punctuation existed in 1980, when the Republican Party containing increased social conservative dominance was elected at the national level. In turn, the punctuation was used to intentionally bring about a conversion effect on the parts of the HHS department dealing with women and children, to defund contraception and fund unscientific abstinence-based education programs. At the same time, the bias of the U.S. pharma industry against considering women's reproductive drugs important and potentially profitable continued. It is clear that Hacker casts the institutionalist concept of drift in a negative light. This analysis also emphasizes that the institutionalist model of layering can be negative or positive, depending on the overall tenor of the government's policy frame. For example, the George W. Bush administration's FDA layered its belated approval of Plan B and RU-486 onto a socially conservative, resistant (but also pro-U.S. pharma) framework. The same president supported the FDA's quick approval of Merck's Gardasil in 2006, when Merck's fortunes were the central issue in the wake of the Vioxx scandal.

The idea that different parts of a polity change at different speeds is highly relevant to and useful for this analysis of the U.S. political structure and its pharma policy. Related to the concepts of layering and conversion, the Clinton administration participated in both negative and positive layering and conversion. The FDA under President Clinton, HHS Secretary Donna Shalala, and FDA Commissioners Kessler and Jane Henney was supportive of Plan B and RU-486, approving both of them on a prescription basis. These actions are defined here as positive layering. The evidence of negative layering was the Personal Responsibility and Work Opportunity Reconciliation Act (PROWRA) of 1996 containing the antichoice provisions related to social security funding of abstinence-only programs. It was passed by a veto-proof majority after the president's veto of a previous version and signed by President Clinton in August 1996. While the FDA in general benefited from a positive pro-choice conversion for the eight years of Bill Clinton's presidency, Congress (under Newt Gingrich) and the conservative House kept the Clinton administration in check.

Other models that enable analysis of the links inside institutions and outside them, yet still within the system of political influence, include those related to social movements and parties. In using the explanations of Tarrow and Burnham, respectively, we can link constituencies outside the FDA to constituencies inside it, party constituencies to Congress, social constituencies to the FDA, and so on. Sidney Tarrow's political process model is discussed since his central factors of movement success and failure are affiliated with the state. They include access to the state, changes in political alignments (such as party control), and support of alliances.[33]

While this book shows mostly that the pharma industry has had much more consistent access to the state than have women in terms of drugs policy, there have been certain points at which state openings occurred and women seized on them accordingly. Such crucial events have included President Franklin Roosevelt's decision to allow contraceptives to be distributed through state health departments, the policies of Presidents Lyndon Johnson and Richard Nixon to provide public funds to underwrite contraceptive distribution, and the role played by President Bill Clinton's administration in helping sell the Marion Merrell Dow company to Hoechst and a reciprocal granting of the RU-486 patent to the U.S.-based Population Council. A feminist response to the Lowi's iron-triangle theory is Stetson's version of an abortion policy triad, containing medical personnel (usually doctors), politicians, and pro-choice social movement organizations.[34] For our purposes, the abortion triad is broadened to include the reproductive choice triad. This triad was represented in the policymaking on public funding of contraception in the 1940s and 1960s and on approval of RU-486 and Plan B by prescription in the Clinton administration. The triad was largely manipulated by Merck and willing politicians to get Gardasil quickly approved by the FDA in 2006 and mandated by some states. For the reproductive choice triad to work well, it has to be embedded within a receptive state, which has largely not been the case since 2000. The FDA under George W. Bush waffled over whether Plan B could be made OTC for certain age groups. That waffling has not disappeared under President Obama's FDA, unfortunately.

Tarrow's theory has much in common with Walter Burnham's theory of cyclical political realignments, where actors who have felt excluded in previous dominant coalitions seize on a dramatic event and frame it so as to engineer new voting patterns and party control of the federal government. This new control, in turn, yields new policy options that had been off the table under previous regimes.[35]

Feminist institutionalism, which is the most important theoretical strand for this book, can incorporate any of the four strands of historical institutionalist theory already discussed. A feminist institutionalist analysis is important to showing why women's reproductive drugs needs were consistently dismissed by the pharma industry through reasons of insufficient profit (the Pill), competition to another drug already sold by Searle (RU-486), not wanting to let women under 17 have state-approved sexual relations (Plan B OTC), and helping Merck by profiting from the fact that women under 17 have sexual relations (Gardasil).

The models of institutional change identified by Streeck and Thelen and Hacker can easily be adapted to feminist purposes.[36] Beyeler and Annesley advance the argument that a "feminist institutionalist perspective on welfare regimes and gender regimes exists . . . even if it has not previously been labelled that way."[37] The notion of what makes feminist institutionalism different from its mainstream counterpart remains undertheorized. Suffice it to say that those of us who consider ourselves feminists and employ institutionalist analyses can be said to be using a feminist institutionalist framework.

The four types of discursive institutionalism described by Lombardo, Meier, and Verloo line up well with some of the gradual historical institutionalist models of Streeck, Thelen, and Hacker. Lombardo et al.'s definition of fixing is consistent with what Streeck et al. term institutional layering. In the Lombardo et al. framework, fixing is defined as "gender equality has been enshrined in legal or political documents and has become recognized as a no longer contested goal."[38] At the other end of the spectrum, bending occurs when gender equality is not at the heart of the debate, but rather is fit into other dominant concepts, such as the example of "strategically framing gender mainstreaming to fit the dominant frame of a given Directorate General."[39] Thus, "bending occurs when the concept of gender equality is adjusted to make it fit some other goal than gender equality itself."[40] The discursive notion of bending would tend to fit well with the politics of either displacement or conversion. The third concept identified by Lombardo et al. is shrinking, whereby gender equality is confined to a particular policy area or a specific interpretation of an issue.[41] Shrinking could accompany the historical institutionalist concept of drift, in which institutions do not keep up with the changing social realities of the external constituency and thus the institution itself, like the type of equality policy it administers, shrinks.

The final concept identified by Lombardo et al. is that of stretching, which "develops a larger meaning (of gender equality) that expands on its previous understanding in a given context."[42] Stretching equality policy to fit other areas of inequality would mean institutionalist conversion or layering of a progressive, rather than regressive manner. Reproductive-rights policy, identified by Mazur as a type of body politics and therefore unique in its application to women, publicizes (makes public) the most private elements of women's lives.[43] She cites Beasley and Bacchi's observation that "citizenship matters for bodies."[44] The consistent denial of women's full citizenship rights to reproductive autonomy in the United States by the market and state is the subject of the rest of the chapters in this book.

PLAN OF THE BOOK

Chapter 2 describes the history of the FDA in the United States since its founding in the early 20th century and the periods of change in the regulatory regimes as described by Ceccoli. Chapter 3 describes the development of the Pill in the United States. It describes how extraordinary efforts by Margaret Sanger, Katherine McCormick, and Gregory Pincus led to the Pill's formulation and convincing Searle to license and market it. In terms of the theories used to explain the case studies, those of Tarrow and Lowi are relevant. So too are historical and feminist discursive institutionalist models. The development of the contraceptive pill is probably the closest example of stretching the concept to cover broad areas of women's equality, for this drug de-linked sex and contraception for the first time. The availability of the Pill from 1960 onward was seized by opponents to fix the notion of women's equality as having been already accomplished. Conversion of the existing system of private provision and funding was changed under the Roosevelt, Nixon, and Johnson administrations for various reasons, when contraception became publicly-funded. The presence of chemical contraception was layered into the nascent contraceptive system of barrier methods.

Chapter 4 describes the pro-choice and antichoice groups on women's reproductive issues in the United States. With the rise of the global demography movement in the 1940s and 1950s and its funding by groups such as the Rockefeller Foundation, contraception and its government funding was on the public discourse in the 1960s. General women's groups such as NOW and specific pro-choice ones such as the NARAL, later changed into the National Abortion Rights Action League, worked from the position that women's rights to control their reproduction would be soundly embedded in national law. The rise of the right-to-life lobby after the unexpectedly broad 1973 U.S. Supreme Court's *Roe v. Wade* decision offered evidence to the contrary. The chief successes of the antichoice or pro-life movement since 1973 have been to return much of the decision-making power to the states over reproductive health and to circumscribe women's pro-choice options through undercutting funding and information about the availability of contraception and abortion. This analysis holds that the most fundamental policy punctuation on women's reproductive rights occurred in 1980 with the election of Ronald Reagan. A long-term conversion of the structures that previously helped women access their rights, mostly headquartered in the national Department of HHS, followed.

Chapter 5 discusses the attempt to get RU-486 imported into the United States, finally successful in the last days of the Clinton administration. Chapter 6 covers the struggle to get Plan B approved for OTC distribution (at least to those 18 and over). Both RU-486 and Plan B were approved by prescription only under the Clinton administration's FDA, late in his second term. RU-486 is likely the most important achievement after the Pill in terms of contributing to women's bodily autonomy. The agreement to approve RU-486 in the United States and to transfer the license to the Population Council was the second example of stretching women's reproductive rights, since RU-486 is the only dedicated medical abortion pill available.

In all three cases after the development of the Pill, the reproductive drugs approved by the FDA were layered onto the existing system. These include RU-486 described in Chapter 5, Plan B described in Chapter 6, and Gardasil discussed in Chapter 7. The layering process includes being added as profit-making entities for their sponsoring companies, and for increasing women's ability to optimize their reproductive health. However, the last case study Gardasil should be treated with caution, since the vast majority of women who need Gardasil are in the Global South. In the Global North, consistent pap smears largely obviate the need for the vaccine. Thus, while the development of the Pill and RU-486 in the United States could be said to have stretched women's autonomy, Plan B is a less likely candidate for that description and Gardasil a most unlikely prospect. As discussed in Chapter 6, the implementation of Plan B availability through state-level studies under collaborative practice frameworks could be viewed as a form of discursive stretching, whereby the prescription age requirement was bypassed.

Overall, it must be said that in the U.S. political system, with its diffusion of powers, most health-care implementation responsibility resting at the state level, and a blatantly for-profit pharmaceutical system, the most common actions to be described under historical institutionalism are layering. The most profound example of conversion, involving all three federal branches, has occurred since 1980 and thus layering since then has tended to be against women's interests. The exception to this was the Clinton-era FDA, in which positive layering occurred. However, the conservative conversion begun in 1980 also betokened drift, in which previously insured women lost insurance coverage and/or public funding for reproductive health care. To relate discursive institutionalist understandings in this instance, we would say that drift has involved shrinking, in which both the discourse and the policy coverage take on a narrower focus. Layering can yield stretching (as in the case of the Pill and RU-486). In terms of the Pill, layering also involved a discursive notion of fixing reproductive rights to a point where they could not be reduced. Under unfriendly administrations, layering can involve shrinking or bending. The instance of Plan B, instituted under a dual regime of prescription-only status for women under 17 and OTC for those 17 and over, would be described as a shrunken discourse, where the right of access is not available to everyone. Finally, the Gardasil case was one of discursive bending, in which U.S. women were manipulated to believe that a wonder drug could achieve something different from routine pap smears.

Given the constraints of the U.S. system of for-profit pharma and diffused political control, it is hypothesized that a true system of discursive stretching, where women in every part of the country have the same access to reproductive drugs under the same conditions as each other, is impossible. The structure of the state-based U.S. health care and insurance systems, layered onto these other realities, in essence confirms that a unified system of reproductive drugs provision is far off into the future, even if President Obama's health care reform law remains in force. These conditions mitigating against a uniform, comprehensive framework of reproductive drugs access is described in the Conclusion, Chapter 8.

NOTES

1. Donald Critchlow, *Intended Consequences: Birth Control, Abortion and the Federal Government in Modern America* (New York: Oxford University, 2001), Chs. 2, 4.

2. Ibid.

3. William Saletan, *Bearing Right: How Conservatives Won the Abortion War* (Berkeley, CA: University of California Press, 2004).

4. Kevin Phillips, *The Emerging Republican Majority* (New York: Anchor, 1970).

5. As accessed from the Guttmacher Institution website, www.guttmacher.org, July 5, 2009.

6. "Preven Contraceptive Kit—the First and Only Emergency Contraceptive Product—Approved by the FDA," Gynetics, September 2, 1998, http://ec.princeton.edu/news/preven.html.

7. Ibid.

8. "Review Summary for Plan B Safety," *Medical Officer Safety Review*, Briefing 4015B1, 2003, http://www.fda.gov/ohrms/dockets/ac/03/briefing/4015B1_12_FDA-Tab%205-1-Medical%20Officer%20Review.htm.

9. "Bush Nominates Mark McClellan to Head the FDA," *Stanford Reporter,* October 2, 2002, http://news.stanford.edu/news/2002/october2/fda-102.html.

10. "Plan B and the Bush Administration," The Emergency Contraception website, http://ec.princeton.edu/pills/planbhistory.html.

11. For example, those who are credited with turning political science back to the study of institutions include James G. March and Johan P. Olsen, "The New Institutionalism: Organizational Factors in Political Life," *The American Political Science Review* 78, no. 2 (1984): 734–49. Others who have emphasized "bringing the state back in" include Peter B. Evans, Dietrich Rueschmeyer, and Theda Skocpol, eds., *Bringing the State Back In* (Cambridge: Cambridge University Press, 1985) and Stephen Skowronek, *Building a New American State: The Expansion of National Administrative Capacities, 1877–1920* (Cambridge: Cambridge University Press, 1982).

12. Daniel Carpenter, *Reputation and Power: Organizational Image and Pharmaceutical Regulation at the FDA* (Princeton, NJ: Princeton University Press, 2010) and *The Forging of Bureaucratic Autonomy: Reputation, Networks and Policy Innovation in Executive Agencies, 1862–1928* (Princeton, NJ: Princeton University Press, 2001).

13. Peter Bachrach and Morton S. Baratz, "Two Faces of Power," *American Political Science Review* 56, no. 4 (December 1962): 947–52.

14. Carpenter, *Reputation and Power,* 15–26.

15. Stephen Ceccoli, *Pill Politics: Drugs and the FDA* (Boulder, CO: Lynne Rienner, 2003). See also Frank Baumgartner and Bryan Jones, *Agendas and Instability in American Politics* (Chicago, IL: University of Chicago Press, 1993) and Frank Baumgartner and Bryan Jones, eds., *Policy Dynamics* (Chicago, IL: University of Chicago Press, 2002).

16. See Theodore J. Lowi, *The End of Liberalism: Ideology, Policy, and the Crisis of Authority* (New York: Norton, 1969) and Melissa Haussman and David Biette, "Buy American or Buy Canadian? Public Procurement Politics and Policy under International Frameworks," in *How Ottawa Spends, 2010–2011: Recession, Realignment and the New Deficit Era,* eds. G. Bruce Doern and Christopher Stoney (Montreal, QC: McGill-Queen's University Press, 2010), 121–49.

17. See especially Amy G. Mazur and Dorothy E. McBride, "Gendering New Institutionalism," in *The Politics of State Feminism: Innovation in Comparative Research* (Philadelphia, PA: Temple University Press, 2010), 217–40; and especially Mona Lena Krook and Fiona Mackay, "Introduction: Gender, Politics and Institutions" and Fiona Mackay, "Towards a Feminist Institutionalism?", in *Gender, Politics and Institutions: Towards a Feminist Institutionalism,* eds. Mona Lena Krook and Fiona Mackay (New York: Palgrave Macmillan, 2011), 1–20 and 181–96, respectively.

18. Mazur and McBride, "Gendering New Institutionalism," 224.

19. Vivien Schmidt, "Discursive Institutionalism: The Explanatory Power of Ideas and Discourse," *Annual Review of Political Science* 11 (2008): 303–26, cited in Mazur and McBride, "Gendering New Institutionalism," 223.

20. Mazur and McBride, "Gendering New Institutionalism," 223; Krook and Mackay, "Introduction: Gender, Politics and Institutions," 9.

21. Barry Weingast, "Rational-Choice Institutionalism," in *Political Science: The State of the Discipline*, eds. Ira Katznelson and Helen Milner (New York: Norton, 2002), 660–92, cited in Krook and Mackay, "Introduction: Gender, Politics and Institutions," 8.

22. Wolfgang Streeck and Kathleen Thelen, eds., *Beyond Continuity: Institutional Change in Advanced Political Economies* (London: Oxford University Press, 2005), 1–39.

23. Streeck and Thelen cite Peter A. Hall and David Soskice, eds., *Varieties of Capitalism: The Institutional Foundations of Comparative Advantage* (Oxford: Oxford University Press, 2001) and Paul Pierson, *Dismantling the Welfare State? Reagan, Thatcher, and the Politics of Retrenchment* (Cambridge: Cambridge University Press, 1994), 5–8.

24. Streeck and Thelen, *Beyond Continuity*, 19.

25. Ibid., 22.

26. Jacob S. Hacker, "Policy Drift: The Hidden Politics of US Welfare State Retrenchment," in Streeck and Thelen, *Beyond Continuity*, 42.

27. Ibid.

28. Hacker, "Policy Drift," 40–83.

29. Ibid., 41.

30. Streeck and Thelen, *Beyond Continuity*, 26.

31. Hacker, "Policy Drift," 42, citing Kathleen Thelen, "How Institutions Evolve: Insights from Comparative Historical Analysis," in *Comparative Analysis in the Social Sciences*, eds. James Mahoney and Dietrich Rueschemeyer (Cambridge: Cambridge University Press, 2003), 208–40.

32. Ibid., 29.

33. Sidney Tarrow, *Power in Movement: Social Movements and Contentious Politics* (Cambridge: Cambridge University Press, 1998).

34. Dorothy M. Stetson, "Abortion Triads and Women's Rights in Russia, the United States, and France," in *Abortion Politics: Public Policy in Cross-Cultural Perspective*, eds. Marianne M. Githens and Dorothy M. Stetson (New York: Routledge, 1996), 97–118.

35. Walter Dean Burnham, *Critical Elections: And the Mainsprings of American Politics* (New York: W. W. Norton and Company, 1971).

36. See the arguments of Michelle Beyeler and Claire Annesley, "Gendering the Institutional Reform of the Welfare State: Germany, the United Kingdom, and Switzerland," in Krook and Mackay, *Gender, Politics and Institutions*, 79–94.

37. Ibid., 80.

38. Emanuela Lombardo, Petra Meier, and Mieke Verloo, eds., *The Discursive Politics of Gender Equality: Stretching, Bending and Policymaking* (Oxon: Routledge, 2009), 3–6.

39. M. A. Pollack and E. Hafner-Burton, "Mainstreaming Gender in the European Union," *Journal of European Public Policy* 7 (2000): 432–56, cited in Lombardo et al., *Discursive Politics*, 6.

40. Lombardo et al., *Discursive Politics*, 5.

41. Ibid.

42. Ibid.

43.   Amy G. Mazur, "Body Politics I: Reproductive Rights Policy," *Theorizing Feminist Policy* (Oxford and New York: Oxford University Press, 2002), Chapter 8, 137–54.

44.   Chris Beasley and Carol Bacchi, "Citizen Bodies: Embodying Citizens—A Feminist Analysis," *International Feminist Journal of Politics* 2, no. 3 (2000): 335–58, cited in Mazur, *Theorizing Feminist Policy,* 137.

2

History of the FDA and Drug Regulation in the United States

This chapter describes the enactment of the food and drug regulatory structure in the United States. In covering the Food and Drug Administration's (FDA) history, the discussion also lays out the degree of political protection for U.S. pharmaceutical companies (called pharma in the discussion) unique to the U.S. political system.

As discussed by Carpenter, the FDA's main source of political capital has been its carefully groomed reputation as a tough drug regulator. Part of this reputation lies in the FDA's image that its drug testing and approval process is the most deliberate in the world. The slowness of the process yields claims by the FDA and its supporters that U.S. consumers and those in other countries who buy FDA-approved drugs are the most protected.[1] As will be shown, the claim that FDA approval's timeline produces enhanced scrutiny and safety is often unsustainable, particularly with regard to women's reproductive drugs.

STRUCTURES FOR POLITICIZATION OF U.S. PHARMA

Measuring the degree and type of politicization in the U.S. pharma policy framework is quite complicated. The complications are found first in the U.S.

health insurance system, which is a patchwork of different state and federal plans, publicly and privately paid. It is disconcerting that in the same country with the highest tolerated drug prices and profits, the largest number of uninsured is also present. The cost controls on U.S. drug prices are minimal, found usually in the public part of the health care system—Medicaid and Medicare.

The FDA is an office within an executive agency (Department of Health and Human Services [HHS]) and it would be logical to expect that it is more permeable to legislative or executive direction than an independent regulatory commission, such as the Interstate Commerce Commission or the Federal Communications Commission. The latter type of agency was set up by Congress to be independent of both private-sector pressure and presidential control in that they either have bipartisan boards of commissioners or in the case of commissions with a chair, the only source of removal by the president is for failing to uphold the oath of office.[2]

Another avenue for the politicization of pharma policy in the United States is, ironically, the set of institutions designed to prevent concentration of power. In many respects, the horizontal and vertical separation of powers has not changed. The interests of the U.S.-based public and private sectors in maintaining the United States as a global financial leader have continued since this argument was used to justify the adoption of the Constitution by the Federalists in 1787. James Madison designed the horizontal separation of powers system so that no one faction could take over all institutions of government. Ironically, the history of this system has been that savvy actors can learn to concentrate on one institution for leverage against the others. Theories that are relevant to the ways in which interest groups or social movements can access power inside U.S. institutions include the following. One is that of the two faces of power envisioned by Bachrach and Baratz in the 1960s. One face is that of highly placed individuals in institutions who can facilitate decision-making. With regard to the first face, that of decision-making, the theories of Theodore Lowi on iron triangles and Sidney Tarrow on the political opportunity structure are relevant. While Lowi's theory is about interest groups and Tarrow's is about social movements, they both consider access to the state to be primary forces explaining the policy successes of groups and movements. In Lowi's theory, interest groups are included in the iron triangle of influence between legislative and executive branches, with the pressure group representing the relevant interest.[3] Too often, pharma policy in the United States has been conducted along this model, with PhRMA—the national lobby group of the pharma industry— being the only nongovernmental officials at the table. Similarly, Tarrow's theory of the political opportunity structure is that when a social movement or representative groups have access to the state, alliances with powerful allies or a shift in political realignments happens, the movement usually affects policy.[4]

The second face of power in Bachrach and Baratz's model is the ability to block decisions from happening.[5] The power to block action may or may not require a change in the structure of one of the branches of government. Instead, a replacement of the actors within the institution may suffice. If the changes are based on replacement within one federal government branch, it is not very likely that the long-term balance of power between Congress and the president will shift. This outcome affirms Madisonian theory. An example of the role of population replacement in the U.S. House is found in the actions of its Republican leadership since it came to power in 2010. The unwillingness of Speaker Boehner to work with President Obama on sweeping social and economic reforms did not require institutional change on the part of Congress, but it was based on a shift in the ideologies of Republicans elected to the House.

Examples of direct shifts in institutional rules since the 1990s affecting this study include those implemented by Congress and the president. With respect to Congress, the relevant change was the rise in omnibus legislation and earmarks in the budget resolution that cannot be taken apart and reviewed by the president.[6] Many social policy changes in the Gingrich–Clinton years, such as changes to the welfare system and the budget for it, were effected through these latter procedures. Regarding the presidency, George W. Bush's implementation of faith-based offices in national agencies, including HHS, has shown institutional change. His changes to the institutions in response to an outside electoral bloc of social conservatives shifted the universe of relevant proposals on women's reproductive rights that got on the political agenda and some of which were funded.

The nature of electoral coalitions within the two-party structure has changed, particularly since the 1970s, with the increasing importance of the growing population of the South and its weight in the electoral college. Those voters have tended to be socially conservative Republicans

The domestic politics of pharma regulations have changed since 1980 to acknowledge the increased power of social conservatives, often from the South, in the Republican coalition. Again, given that there are constants and changes in U.S. political institutions and pharma policies, an ongoing theme is that pharma and the U.S. government work together to protect pharma's interests. Where social conservative rhetoric can be used to demonstrate the riskiness of ventures on women's reproductive drugs, companies will use it. This study's interpretation of the social conservative theme is that it is used to justify pharma's laser-like focus on the bottom line. However, change has also been seen in the U.S. pharma policy's history since social conservatives have been more dominant on the U.S.

political scene at certain times than at others. The two times, in particular, have been the late 19th century since the 1873 promulgation of the federal Comstock Act and since the election of Ronald Reagan to the presidency in 1980.

Finally, another example of historical continuity in the U.S. government is that the FDA, like so much of the rest of the structure, continues to be dominated by men. The first female FDA commissioner, Dr. Jane Henney, served two years during the Clinton administration (1999–2001), having been one of the first two women deputy commissioners appointed to the FDA in 1991—along with Deputy Commissioner Carol Scheman the same year. The second female FDA commissioner, Dr. Margaret Hamburg, took up her post in May 2009.[7] By contrast, the first female Cabinet secretary in the United States was Frances Perkins, appointed by President Roosevelt to Labor in 1933. Until the representation of women with power to effect decision-making in Congress, the executive branch (including the FDA), and pharma increases, it is most likely that pharma policy in the United States will be concerned only with a narrow definition of the bottom line. Needless to say, the frame does not include women's needs in a manner to increase their autonomy in society.

THEORETICAL FRAMEWORK OF THE CHAPTER

In terms of the theoretical perspectives used in this chapter, the iron-triangle theory of Lowi, Tarrow's political process model, and Burnham's realignment theories of U.S. party politics are all relevant.[8] These views help us to describe the most important feature of U.S. prescription drug policy over time, which is its constant overlooking of women's needs. They also help us understand women's varying degrees of access to the state in terms of pharma policy, most notably during the Johnson, Nixon, Ford, and Clinton administrations.

Ceccoli's theories of FDA adaptation are based on the rather abrupt discontinuities envisioned by Baumgartner and Jones.[9] In particular, he refers to policy punctuations in response to certain focusing events from John Kingdon's theory. Carpenter's historical theory can be related to Ceccoli's use of Baumgartner and Jones's punctuated equilibrium model. Carpenter adapted the Bachrach and Baratz two-faces-of-power model to include a third, that of reputational power, which can be traced to actors' ability to shape the political discourse. In crucial instances, Carpenter suggests that a combination of actors inside the FDA worked with some citizen groups to force reluctant presidents, including Franklin D. Roosevelt and John Kennedy, to strengthen the FDA's regulatory powers. The discursive punctuations brought about parts of the legislation that the FDA actors wished to have and also enabled the FDA to keep burnishing its image as the world's chief pharma regulator.[10] In short, Ceccoli's and Carpenter's views are combined in this study to talk about policy punctuations and how reputational power can be co-opted against women's reproductive health questions. It also must be noted that Carpenter specifically rejects the notion of sharp policy punctuations, described as "binary before and after narratives."[11] It is possible to combine the two accounts by emphasizing what is new in distinct policy punctuations, while also emphasizing the possibility of institutional and policy continuation across the time periods.

This book separates the development of policy and rhetoric on women's reproductive pharma needs into two policy punctuations. The first policy punctuation, from the 1960s until 1980, was largely not driven by feminist interests, nor did it have a significant amount of women in federal office. However, women were helped in a few distinct ways. The first policy system on women's reproductive matters was an expansionist one with its roots in the Social Security Act of 1935, but the height of activity started in 1960, when the FDA approved the Pill for contraceptive purposes, and lasted through *Roe v. Wade* in 1973. In between these two events, Congress passed Title X of the Public Health Services Act to publicly fund contraception in 1970 and pro-contraception decisions occurred at the Supreme Court.[12] The FDA's approval of the Pill was significant in that it was the first drug to be recommended to healthy people for the long term. It was helpful that Presidents Johnson and Nixon supported public funding for contraception globally and in the United States. Their support derived heavily from the access to the state that demographers had in the 1960s. These scientists came armed with studies of population rate increases around the world, particularly in developing countries. One world event relevant to the Rockefeller Foundation's support of such research was the misnamed 1959–1961 Great Leap Forward in China during which millions starved.[13] Demographers had willing ears in Washington in the 1960s. In the first period on women's reproductive policy from 1960 to 1973, the interests of U.S. women in having access to publicly-funded contraception was achieved through substantive representation. This type of representation was a response to the frame of global pressures felt by large populations.

The second policy punctuation on women's reproductive rights has happened in the United States since 1980. It started with a Republican-led attack on the practices of government funding during the first policy period. The goal during the second policy period has been to deny a national system of contraception and abortion access, through restricting funding and allowing states to restrict abortion provision in various ways. The two major Supreme Court cases concerning abortion during the second policy period were the 1989 *Webster* and 1992 *Casey* decisions.[14] The abstinence-based education legislation began in 1981 under Senators Jeremiah Denton and Orrin Hatch. The Clinton years were divided on public health and women, since Congressional control was divided in those years, including the 20th century's most socially conservative House. While the Clinton administration was helpful on RU- 486 and Plan B, the Gingrich-led Congress in 1996 enlarged the framework of abstinence-based services that was fully realized under the George W. Bush administrations. Control of the FDA and HHS was given to social conservatives from 2000 to 2008. While the Obama administration and the one session of Democratic control of both houses of Congress worked to change some of the second policy period's negativity toward women, policy remnants are still in place. These continuations include the abstinence-based funding stream in the Social Security Act, although greatly reduced, and the faith-based office in the White House.

Historical and discursive institutionalisms are important in showing how different parties in power since 1900 used different ideas to streamline or try to block pharma dominance at the FDA. At some points, additions to FDA regulations would fit under the layering model described by Streeck and Thelen and Hacker. As described by Wolfgang Streeck and Kathleen Thelen, and Jacob Hacker, layering occurs when actors change parts of the institution that they find still open to change, rather than the parts that have been closed off to change through path dependency, wherein previously established rules and structures show lock-in effects. Drift is used to describe a situation whereby an institution does not keep up with changing times and the institution's outside constituency actually loses coverage because of this; and conversion, where institutions are "redirected to new goals or purposes."[15] As described by Hacker regarding the U.S. health insurance system, the creation and modification of the FDA is also explained by theories of drift and conversion. The applicability of the conversion model will be clear throughout this analysis, since socially conservative Republican control of the presidency, the FDA, and Congress yielded even worse changes to the drug policy regarding women than the norm of pharma indifference. The reliance on conversion theory pairs well with that on policy or institutional drift, for explaining other changes in the pharma policy system concerning women. Socially conservative Republican control of national office—unlike the public funding of contraception under the Johnson and Nixon administrations—yielded policy and institutional drift at HHS. The evidence of drift is found in dropping many U.S. women—especially the poor, teenaged, and marginalized—from health care plans covering contraceptive and abortion services. At the same time, purported social conservatives such as Rick Perry were willing to allow Medicaid coverage for Texas women for Gardasil shots, but not abortions. These examples show the power of combining conversion and drift models particularly with regard to women as parts of feminist historical institutionalism.

THE FOR-PROFIT NATURE OF U.S. PHARMA

The for-profit nature of the U.S. pharma industry, particularly the huge companies at the top of the chain, enables it to claim that it only considers the financial feasibility of drugs and not their social implications.

The cost-benefit analysis performed by U.S. drug companies works from the end of the equation back to the beginning.[16] Each company must figure out which blockbuster drugs with annual sales of at least 1 billion dollars are due to expire within the 20-year patent frame, and then assess where other potential blockbusters to replace them are located in the company's R&D pipeline. For a U.S. pharma company to survive, it needs a blockbuster on the market every three years. As noted by Ravenscraft and Long, the U.S.-based pharma industry (the largest global market) found itself facing a crisis of available long-term funding in the early 1990s. As they note, "in 1993, there were 21 billion-dollar-per-year patents on the market and most were slated to expire in 2000 . . . yet not a single new drug was expected to reach this blockbuster status during the same time period."[17]

POLITICAL PROTECTION FOR U.S. PHARMA

U.S. drugs receive 20 years' patent protection in the United States. Any foreign-owned drug that could be placed in competition with a U.S.-owned drug either under review by the FDA or on the market also has to go through FDA review. Thus, it is basically impossible for a foreign-crafted and foreign-approved drug to jump the pipeline ahead of a U.S.-based drug. Since the 1848 Drug Importation Act was renewed in various legislative and administrative laws, foreign-made is officially treated by the FDA and the U.S. drug industry as unsafe and impure, requiring the same FDA testing as any U.S.-based drugs. The 1938 Food, Drug, and Cosmetic Act (FDCA) governing the FDA states that no foreign drug or copy of an American drug will be allowed on the U.S. market until it has passed FDA approval.[18] This import regulation was strengthened in the Kefauver amendments to the FDCA in 1962 and repeated in the Administrative Procedure Act of 1946, an act governing the administration of U.S. agencies. Any U.S.-based company that wants to license a foreign company's drug for U.S. sales also must go through the FDA. Indeed, as Chicoine has aptly pointed out, part of the comparative slowness in drug approval in the United States is that the FDA requires data from U.S.-based studies at all points before marketing, while other countries such as Britain will rely on foreign-generated data.[19]

The fact that drugs from non-U.S.-based companies must get FDA approval before being sold in the United States gives the FDA great power as a gatekeeper, as noted by Carpenter.[20] The irony is that foreign-tested and foreign-approved drugs are often safely used on the global market for decades before the FDA allows them into the United States, as was true with RU-486 and Plan B. As part of the iron triangle in pharma policymaking, the FDA protects U.S. pharma as much as it regulates them.

U.S. pharma industries are consistently at or near the top of the annual Fortune 500 list. Pfizer has been the top performer in the global market since the late 1990s, and Merck has usually been second during that time. These market positions are related to this analysis in that Pfizer acquired Searle, the number one maker of birth-control pills in the United States in 2003, and Merck makes Gardasil. A 2009 report on the Fortune 500 list by CNN Money numbered the sectors by profits received as a percentage of overall revenues in 2008. Network and communications came in first at 20.4 percent, the Internet second at 19.4 percent, pharma was third at 19.3 percent, and medical devices fourth at 16.3 percent.[21] Marcia Angell, MD, senior lecturer at Harvard Medical School and the first woman editor-in-chief of the prestigious *New England Medical Journal,* observed that, "in 2002,the top 10 drug companies in the United States had a median profit margin of 17%, compared with only 3.1% for all the other industries on the Fortune 500 list . . . those 10 companies made more in profits that year than the other 490 companies put together." She also wryly notes that there are far more drug industry lobbyists in the United States than there are members of Congress.[22]

LEGISLATIVE CHANGES TO THE U.S. DRUG APPROVAL PROCESS

Institutional continuities and changes may be found in detailing the history of the FDA's forerunners from 1906 onward. Ceccoli believes that in different periods of time, the FDA has pitted avoiding Type I errors of being overly cautious and Type II errors of rushing drugs to market against each other.[23] For the purposes of feminist institutionalism, we can suggest that the layering of more policy tools onto the FDA's enabling legislation during the 20th century had the potential to help women. The relevant tools included ways for the FDA to scrutinize and keep unsafe drugs off the market. In most instances, except in the most recent one concerning Gardasil, these policy tools worked as intended. In other instances, such as with RU-486 and Plan B, the policy tools were misappropriated to stall safe drugs from being put on the U.S. market.

There are five major pieces of legislation to cover, with some narrower clarifying amendments taking place in between them as will be noted. The centerpiece of FDA regulation remains the 1938 FDCA, the main regulatory framework for the U.S. pharma policy. There were two important sets of changes to the 1938 law, the 1962 Kefauver amendments and the 1992 Prescription Drug User Fee Act (PDUFA).[24] It is also vital to describe the rise of the U.S. generics regime as helped along by the 1984 Drug Price Competition and Patent Term Restoration Act, commonly known as the Hatch-Waxman Act.

DEVELOPMENTS BEFORE THE 1938 FDCA

In 1820, the first U.S. pharmacopoeia, known as the National Formulary, was published.[25] According to the FDA website, the first person appointed to monitor food safety was Lewis Beck in the patent office in 1848, whose functions were then moved over to the Bureau of Chemistry in the Department of Agriculture in 1862.[26] In the mid-19th century, due to a lack of strong import controls, the United States was the recipient of the "world's counterfeit, contaminated, diluted and decomposed drug materials."[27] Congress responded to this with the 1848 Drug Importation Act.

In 1862, the agriculture department's chemistry division became the main locus of food-safety measures and those related to drugs. The chemistry division was said to have the only well-functioning laboratory in the capital until the 20th century.[28] On one hand, much social change was occurring at the middle of the 19th century that showed a role for strengthened public-health mechanisms. Some of the indicators were population shifts from rural to urban areas, lack of proper sanitation in the cities, and the sustained usage of toxic additives in foods.[29] Interests in the drug and health industries also started to organize. Notable among them was the American Medical Association (AMA) in 1847, and the start of the public-health movement. Other, less savory formalization was also taking place with the establishment of storefronts and traveling operations to sell quack medicines.[30]

The first significant policy punctuation in FDA history is identified by Ceccoli as the 1906 Pure Food and Drugs Act (PFDA), and a discursive institutionalist frame is applicable. The director of the agriculture department's chemistry division was scientist Harvey Wiley, who had been appointed in 1883. Ceccoli believes that the 1887 Hatch Act helped Wiley to make the case for strengthening the division. Part of the Hatch Act provided federal funding for agricultural experimental stations to be set up at state land-grant colleges and universities.[31]

Harvey Wiley was an innovator, a coalition builder, and in the social movement literature parlance, a movement entrepreneur.[32] Since the early division's remit was based on a discipline (chemistry), its rationale was based on "finding a problem to solve."[33] In his role as coalition builder, Wiley brought in various interests including those from the consumer protection sector and the Woman's Christian Temperance Union (WCTU) to testify for anti-adulteration legislation in Congress. The election of pro-market Progressive President Theodore Roosevelt in 1900 strengthened the case for a stronger national regulatory framework for the food and agriculture industries.

Congress passed the Meat Inspection Act and the PFDA in 1906.[34] The PFDA focused mostly on regulation of the food industry but also mandated the chemistry bureau to take adulterated, misbranded, or unsafe drugs from public distribution. The standard measurement would continue to be the 1820 U.S. pharmacopoeia, the National Formulary. The policy period begun by the PFDA's passage in 1906 is termed by Eisner as a market regime of regulation, where national government instruments were formulated to gently correct the market, based on the ethos of competition.[35] On the positive side, the chemistry bureau's budget appropriation was increased fivefold and its staff increased fourfold between 1906 and 1908.[36]

In 1930, the Bureau of Chemistry was renamed the FDA. The notorious example of the 1906 PFDA's loopholes is found in the Sulfanilamide Elixir case. Massengill was a local company started in Tennessee by Dr. Samuel Massengill. The elixir contained a highly toxic combination of diethylene glycol (DEG, used for industrial coolants) and sulfa. Sulfa drugs had been recently found to be effective antibacterial agents, used on many including one of President Roosevelt's sons for a strep infection. The problematic element was DEG, which had not been tested on humans. Despite this, hundreds of bottles were sent out to distributors, pharmacists, and physicians mainly in Mississippi and Oklahoma. The elixir was sold for use mainly for gonorrhea, sore throats, and other infections. Dr. Frances Oldham Kelsey, a pharmacologist, had tested DEG on animals in a previous, unrelated study and found it to be unsafe. The elixir's labeling also contravened the 1906 legislation, since an elixir was required to contain alcohol under the National Drug Formulary and the elixir did not. Malfeasance by the company continued. Until the deaths of more than 100 people were brought to the FDA's attention, the government did not start prosecuting the company and its founder. After a trial, the Massengill company paid the highest fine to date under the 1906 PFDA (16,800 dollars in 1938, equivalent to about 253,000 dollars in 2009). However, Dr. Massengill received no jail time and was elected chamber of commerce president for his town of Bristol, Tennessee in 1939. The chamber of commerce had been his staunch defender.[37]

In the 1930s, those unsatisfied with the 1906 legislation included the director of the FDA, Walter Campbell—its first attorney in the post—and Rexford Tugwell—the assistant secretary of agriculture—who was from early on known as an anticorporate man.[38] Campbell and Tugwell drafted model legislation in 1933 to increase the FDA's powers over the enforcement of false advertising and to require proof of safety before drug approval.[39] The League of Women Voters and Eleanor Roosevelt were strong participants in helping to focus Congress's will in this matter.[40]

Another consciousness-raising event around this horrific failure was that an Oklahoma mother, who had lost her nine-year-old in the typically slow, painful death ascribed to the elixir, wrote a letter about the tragedy to President Roosevelt. It is generally thought that the letter was given to Eleanor Roosevelt, since it also found its way into the press. This speculation is based on the idea that since Eleanor Roosevelt was a public-interest crusader generally and a birth-control supporter specifically, she was very likely the link to the press. The legislation, stalled for years, was passed within six months of the Massengill judgment.[41] Carpenter states that the backers of the FDCA in effect kept the sulfanilamide disaster in the press, so as to force Congress and the president to support the legislation.[42] Carpenter suggests that the proponents' highlighting this disaster was a discursive strategy related to two faces of power, the gatekeeping power, and the desire to enhance the FDA's reputational power. Of course, these powers would cycle back in a feedback loop, where reputational power would enable more decision and non–decision-making power, and these powers if used correctly would polish the FDA's image. Carpenter notes the selective process at work in framing the victims of sulfanilamide. While black men with sexually transmitted diseases (STDs) were the most numerous recipients of the elixir, the story was based on bringing case histories of married white women to the fore.[43]

1938 FEDERAL FOOD, DRUG, AND COSMETIC ACT (FDCA)

There were many crucial parts of the 1938 federal FDCA that the FDA had supported.[44] One of the strongest parts of the act was to require proof of safety by companies before the FDA would approve the drug and allow it to be marketed. Crucial to this passage was the FDA's ability to withhold these drugs from interstate commerce. Before 1938, companies had been able to get FDA approval prior to human testing and could then start marketing the drug. One very strange loophole included in the FDCA was that it required the FDA to deny an application within 60 days, unless a postponement for a maximum of another 2 months was given. If neither procedure happened, the drug was automatically approved.[45]

The 1938 legislation also specified that false or misleading product labels were illegal. The FDA was only given power over drug labeling, not advertising, which went to the Federal Trade Commission. New powers given to the FDA in 1938 included the power to inspect pharma factories and to take a drug off the market if shown to be unsafe.[46] The 1938 act also introduced the category of prescription drugs. This new process vaulted doctors into the central position as connector between patient and pharma (or provider and purchaser). Since pharma, doctors, and hospitals in the United States are in the private sector, the reinforcement of private-sector influence from the start of pharma regulation is important to note. The 1951 Durham-Humphrey Amendment to the FDCA defined which drugs would be in the prescription category.

The embedding of new regulatory powers in the FDA, especially those to require proof of safety before approval and marketing, was heavily contested by U.S. pharma. The legislation that passed in 1938 had been considered in various formats since 1936.[47] Carpenter notes that the FDCA provisions were the death knell of the U.S. patent medicines industry.[48] One huge obstacle to the FDCA was that the 75th U.S. House elected in 1936 was comprised of more conservative Southern Democrats than its predecessor. While it was Democratically controlled, the House put many obstacles in the way of the New Deal legislation. Part of the conversion effect in the 75th Congress was the rise of the "Conservative Coalition and its hostile takeover of the House Rules Committee."[49]

As the FDA has gained increased powers to regulate pharma since 1938, Carpenter notes that legislative changes to the FDA's jurisdiction have enabled the U.S. pharma industry to expand its power from simply a producer to that of sponsor.[50] Carpenter also states that a firm's profits depend on its reputation for negotiating with the FDA and with competitor firms.

Thus, he suggests that the FDA holds some power over drug firms by being able to affect their reputation and their repeat chances of success when they come before the agency with future drug requests. An executive with an unnamed pharma company wrote in the *PharmExec* magazine in 2007 that:

> It's common knowledge that the speed with which FDA approves drugs goes in cycles. The regulatory barriers to approval move like a pendulum, rising and falling based on pressure from Congress, advocates, and, yes, even industry. "There is no constant, quantifiable bar for either safety or efficacy," said Ken Kaitlin, who heads the Tufts Center for the Study of Drug Development.[51]

The passage of the 1938 FDCA made a difference between the outcomes of the sulfanilamide case of the 1930s and the thalidomide case of the 1960s. The actions of drug companies, doctors, and pharmacists were no different in the thalidomide case from the sulfanilamide one. Given the changes in the law in 1938 to require safety before FDA approval and then drug marketing, and a courageous new employee of the FDA, thalidomide's spread in the United States was curtailed, although not completely. The actions of Richardson-Merrell skirted a very thin border of illegality in the thalidomide case. Dr. Frances Kelsey, who joined the FDA in 1960 and ultimately became chief of the Division of New Drugs and then director of the Division of Scientific Investigation, refused to issue approval for thalidomide. She was the newest medical officer, and the thalidomide NDA (New Drug Application) was assigned to her.[52] Upon receiving her M.D. in 1950, Kelsey had worked as an editorial associate at the *Journal of the American Medical Association* (*JAMA*). She stated that

> I soon learned . . . that good scientists are almost invariably good writers and that poor writing is almost invariably a sign of poor science. . . . When I came to the Food and Drug Administration . . . I found that many of the studies in support of the safety of the new drugs were done by investigators whose work had not been accepted for publication in JAMA.[53]

Thalidomide was used as an antidepressant and sleep aid in 46 countries starting in 1957. While Richardson-Merrell asserted that all trials of the drug showed that it was safe, new data was starting to come in. By 1961, numerous cases of birth defects were reported from Canada, Germany, and other European countries. According to the National Institutes of Health, "Dr. Helen Taussig learned of the tragedy from one of her students and traveled to Europe to investigate. By testifying before the Senate, Taussig was able to help Kelsey ban thalidomide in the United States for good."[54] In the United States, Richardson-Merrell had given out "more than 2.5 million thalidomide tablets in 'clinical trials' to 1267 physicians who gave them to 20, 000 patients."[55] Kelsey returned the NDA to the company within the required 60-day period. Different numbers have been given as to the number of families who settled with the pharma company in the United States but they are usually estimated at less than 20.[56]

Doctors Kelsey and Taussig were both female pioneers in the medical field and distinguished scientists and doctors. Dr. Kelsey was given the highest civilian honor, the President's Award for Distinguished Federal Civil Service in 1962, the second woman to receive the honor. Before she became active in the thalidomide issue, the cardiologist Helen Taussig had identified the cause of blue baby syndrome as inadequate blood flow to the lungs and developed a new form of cardiac surgery to correct it. She was one of the first women to achieve the status of full professor at the Johns Hopkins Medical School. She was given the Presidential Medal of Freedom by Lyndon Johnson in 1964.[57]

It is not surprising that the politician who chose to shepherd through significant changes to the 1938 FDCA was Estes Kefauver (D-TN). Since being elected to the Senate in 1948, Estes Kefauver had chaired the high-profile antiracketeering subcommittee, then became interested in the anticompetitive behavior of the steel and auto industries.[58] His attention then shifted to the similar types of inflationary behavior practiced by the U.S. pharma industry. In 1960, a poll showed that 65 percent of the U.S. public thought that prescription prices were too high.[59] Kefauver worked on a bill to improve pharma practices, including adding the criterion of effectiveness to safety required by the FDA and to license pharma companies under standards developed by the FDA.

Kefauver's other crucial goal, resisted heavily by pharma for decades, was to encourage the development of a U.S. generic drug system. The envisioned outcomes were to lower prices and lessen the influence of a few large pharma companies. In promoting generics, Kefauver wanted to change patenting for the most-profitable new molecular entities. They are both the statistically smallest number of drugs and the most heavily protected by patents. The senator proposed a system in which other drug companies could pay a small royalty to the firm that originally developed the drug, three years after patent protection had been acquired. Kefauver also proposed to remove the far larger universe of medications colloquially known as the me-too drugs from patent protection entirely. Another component of the proposal equally distasteful to industry was to raise incentives for the FDA to approve and physicians to offer generic drugs to consumers, giving the FDA the "capacity to declare generic drugs to be of equivalent quality and purity as trade name drugs."[60] The proposals were contained in S. 1552, reported from a Judiciary subcommittee in Spring 1961.

Quickly, the AMA opposing the efficacy requirement and pharma opposing any loosening of patent protections reached their reliable Senate allies, Republicans Everett Dirksen (R-IL) and Roman Hruska (R-NB). As Carpenter notes, Kefauver's bill was defanged when it came out of the subcommittee and never left the Judiciary Committee.[61]

The denial of FDA approval for thalidomide sales in the United States is described by Ceccoli as the focusing event that pushed Congress to pass the Kefauver amendment. Carpenter describes the impetus as a more broad and gradual series of events. Carpenter shows that some within the FDA had pushed for an efficacy-based standard in the 1950s.[62] His point is also that there is a gradual development of standards within the FDA over time that get used informally before they are legislatively enacted. Kelsey's appropriation of the effectiveness criterion was one such example. Unlike Ceccoli, Carpenter identifies the publicity over thalidomide, facilitated by Kefauver's subcommittee, as the focusing event rather than the thalidomide issue itself. The reason for making the distinction is that years elapsed between global awareness of the issue, withdrawal of the application to license distribution in the United States, and the U.S. public's knowledge.[63] Even in February 1962, one month before Merrell, the hopeful U.S. licensee for the drug pulled the application from the FDA, a *Time* magazine editorial doubted that the 3,000 babies said to be affected could all be explained by the mother's exposure to thalidomide.[64]

The Kefauver amendments changed the existing language from requiring a new drug to be safe to get FDA approval to requiring it to be effective as well. This provision required retroactive testing of all drugs approved since 1938 for effectiveness.[65] Another major improvement was the requirement of informed consent for clinical trials in the United States.[66] The United Nations had adopted such a mandate in the 1940s, but Congress and the FDA had not incorporated it into domestic practice.

The 1962 legislation strengthened the FDA's role by increasing the first waiting period for the drug application to 90 days from 60 days. The 1962 framework added a few more steps into the approvals process, including that the secretary of HHS (where the FDA was moved in 1980) has 180 days from the company's NDA filing to either approve it, "convince the applicant to voluntarily delay it," or schedule a hearing for the company on its application to take place within 4 months, after which the secretary must render a decision in 3 months.[67]

The most important part of the 1962 legislation was the addition of the efficacy requirement before drugs could be approved, meaning that companies had to prove both efficacy and safety. Efficacy was rather loosely defined, as firms having to prove that the drug behaved the way the manufacturer said it would. The Kefauver language calls for substantial evidence of safety and efficacy, found in two clinical trials, before allowing approval. Carpenter notes that the efficacy standard was pushed both by Kefauver in Congress and also in model legislation submitted to it by the FDA's Bureau of Medicines in 1960 and 1961.[68] Carpenter states that the president and Congress "willfully left many concepts undefined in the Kefauver legislation, including: new drug; efficacy; adequate, well-controlled; investigations, and scientific training and experience."[69]

Another requirement of the Kefauver legislation, quickly subverted by both pharma and doctors, was the full disclosure rule on labels, followed a few years later by a package insert detailing the drug's safety and efficacy. While this insert was ostensibly for the benefit of the patient, it was really directed toward the doctors.[70] In 1969, an editorial in *JAMA* noted that the FDA did not participate in writing pamphlet inserts into packaging and leaving the labeling and insert writing up to the pharma companies themselves, who also paid for the inserts. Thus, the full disclosure of how to use the prescription and information on potential side effects was left up to the companies.

U.S. doctors clearly prize their autonomy in prescription writing, which was given to them through the FDCA. Doctors complained that informing patients more would interfere with the doctor–patient relationship. Second, doctors claimed that the government was trying to interfere in this relationship. Pharma and physician arguments coincided here in an interesting way, where companies argued that according to the 1938 FDCA, prescription drugs were only to be issued on a physician's recommendation. Companies also stated that opening up this relationship by requiring more information for patients was tantamount to interfering with the delicate nature of the physician–patient relationship. A likely related concern for the companies was that unless otherwise prohibited, physicians can write prescriptions for off-label purposes. In this manner, a single drug is prescribed for many uses, not just the conditions indicated on the label.

Most in the United States approved of the Kefauver amendments as a necessary set of changes to ensure drug consistency and safety. By the 1970s, the U.S.-based pharma industry started complaining about the new law. Claims were made that the new additional layer of FDA review required by the 1962 amendments dramatically slowed the pace of development, resulting in 25 fewer drugs being approved per year. The drug industry complained that the new efficacy requirement forced it to spend much more on research and development.[71] One way found around this by the companies running contraceptive studies outside the United States in the 1960s was to solicit the support of foundations such as Packard, Rockefeller, Pathfinder, and the Population Council.

Congress responded to these criticisms by passing new legislation tilted more in pharma's favor. The laws included the 1983 Orphan Drug Act, to give tax deductions and exclusive marketing rights to manufacturers willing to undertake the expense of developing drugs for treating rare diseases. Another was the implementation of the FDA's compassionate use program to allow access to drugs not yet approved on an individual basis, where those with a serious illness have not been helped by other drugs.[72]

HATCH-WAXMAN AND PATENT CHANGES FOR GENERICS

The next major set of changes to U.S. pharma policies was the Hatch-Waxman Act of 1984, the Drug Price Competition and Patent Term Restoration Act. While this legislation amended both the 1938 FDCA and the various iterations of the federal Patent Act, it also accomplished some unrealized aims of the Kefauver amendments. Overall, the idea was to promote the development of nonbrand-name (generic) competitors to brand-name drugs and to stimulate pharma research in that area. Generics manufacturers would have to demonstrate the bioequivalence, not exact sameness, to a molecule of an already-approved drug. This would take place in a new process, the Abbreviated New Drug Application (ANDA). The firm making the generic drug would also have to file notice regarding its targeted patent drug. All of the patented and FDA-approved drugs are listed in what is called the FDA's Orange Book. Generics manufacturers were given the right to file challenges to the patent term obtained by the original brand-name drug. In a balancing act, patent owners were given the right to force the FDA to stay an ANDA for a month if the patent owner filed suit within 45 days of receiving notice of the generic challenge to its patent. Generics companies also have rights during this period, in which they themselves receive six months' protection of their drug application from any other generics trying to cut in on the early adapter's slice of the market pie. Not coincidentally, the first generic company gets to charge a higher price during this six-month exclusivity period.[73] In addition, Rumore notes that before Hatch-Waxman, only 35 percent of top-selling brand-name drugs had generic competition, and since then generics compete with virtually all of those drugs.[74]

It is also the case that ANDAs have risen significantly, particularly since 1998. A potential reason for this is the consolidation within the U.S. pharma industry between 1994 and 1996, discussed later in the chapter. The balancing act intention of the Hatch-Waxman Act was to get generic drugs to market faster, to promote pharma research at the brand companies, and to give brand-name companies extra patent coverage for the period of time lost during their FDA applications process.[75] While the generic part has certainly worked well, numerous criticisms have also surfaced. The critiques have concerned frivolous patent-protection lawsuits by brand companies to extend their patents and generic brand-name company collusion in the development and timing of ANDAs for generics companies.[76]

CHANGES SINCE THE LATE 1980S

The FDA instituted an expedited review process in 1988. Under the expedited process, the FDA can help set up clinical trials and waive the Phase III trial requirement for approvals. The 1988 legislation is widely viewed as a result of activity by politically savvy lay actors and doctors wanting to speed up the availability of drugs to combat HIV/AIDS. Organizations such as ACT-UP (the AIDS Coalition to Unleash Power) and Project Inform were leaders in this effort.[77] One account claims that the HIV/AIDS crisis starting in the early 1980s was the "first social movement in the US to accomplish the large-scale conversion of disease 'victims' into activists-experts."[78] Epstein notes that "AIDS activists entered deeply into all aspects of the drug review process."[79] In 1992, the 1988 legislation was broadened to allow unapproved drugs to reach the market before complete effectiveness, as required under the 1962 law, had been proven.[80]

Another set of events changing the FDA emphasis by adding timeliness to safety was based on the Reagan ethos of 1980–1988. An important concept was that of marketizing the way that the bureaucracy worked. One example was President Reagan's Executive Order 12291, allowing the Office of Management and Budget (OMB) to "perform a cost-benefit analysis on and therefore screen all government regulations."[81] This new procedure was required of the FDA commissioner, who had to "secure OMB approval of his prepared written remarks when testifying before Congress." Former FDA commissioner Dr. David Kessler wrote that this described policy of deregulation meant that "sometimes relatively low-level desk officers could thwart regulations proposed by a Cabinet secretary."[82]

As FDA commissioner, Dr. David Kessler was adept at making the case for improved pre-approval review times for drugs. The 1992 PDUFA was a solution to the shortfall of FDA funding and drug approval lags by shifting costs to the pharma companies. In fiscal year 2003 figures, PDUFA levied a fee of 100,000 dollars on each company for an NDA to pay for hiring more FDA reviewers. This fee was originally suggested in a 1971 General Accounting Office report. By the 1990s when the U.S. pharma industry was shown that it lost 10 million dollars in sales every month a drug approval was delayed, it participated more in the PDUFA system.[83] By 2006, studies showed that PDUFA revenue alone accounted for 42 percent of the FDA drug-approval budget in the FDA's Center for Drug Evaluation and Research and about 20 percent of overall FDA revenues.[84] A doctor at Harvard Medical School has noted that "it is unusual for a regulatory agency to derive such a large portion of its revenue from the industry it regulates," and others have claimed that the FDA has been turned into the government relations arm of the pharma industry.[85]

By the late 1990s, drug approval wait times had been changed to be among the shortest in the world.[86] Similarly, by 2000, "drugs were being approved in less than half the time of a decade ago."[87] Finally, while up until the late 1980s, the percentage of drugs whose first market was the United States was only 20 percent, by 1996–1998 it had gone up to nearly half (49%). The combined goals of speeding up reviews and helping the U.S.-based drug industry seemed to work for many drugs by the 1990s (but not RU-486 or Plan B). For example, as noted by Hollander, Pfizer's Viagra was approved in less than six months of its application to the FDA on March 27, 1998.[88] It only reached blockbuster status of more than 1 billion dollars annually in 2010, which negates pharma's argument that it only supports drugs based on their profitability.

CONCLUSION

Based on the changes of 1988 and 1992 allowing expedited review and marketing of drugs in their preapproval stages, it is clear that the FDA has the power it needs to expedite drugs when it so chooses. The reasons behind it not doing so on the Plan B and RU-486 approval requests do not put the agency in a good light and demonstrate that the ability to politicize the drug-approval process in the United States has continued unabated.

In addition to the relevance of the theories of Tarrow, Baumgartner and Jones, Ceccoli, and Carpenter in this chapter, institutionalist theories have shown explanatory power. In particular, the layering process alluded to by Streeck and Thelen and Hacker was important for tracing presidential and Congressional willingness to strengthen the FDA's enforcement powers from 1906 to 1962. The conversion of the FDA's processes is shown in two sets of examples since the 1970s. The first is in pharma's agitation starting in the 1970s for FDA approval processes to be shortened. The other example shows the conversion of the FDA's goal to social conservative ends, embedded in the New Right's goals since 1980 for fundamentally shifting HHS and its programmatic funding. That example also implies drift, since the risk pool of women covered by HHS and FDA programs shrunk under the social conservative watch, with the exception of Gardasil, mandated to help Merck's fortunes.

Discursive institutionalism was also important across the different periods, first used by reformers through 1962 and then by pharma, as it claimed to be unfairly burdened by FDA slowness. In terms of feminist institutionalism, Eleanor Roosevelt, Drs. Frances Kelsey and Helen Taussig, the WCTU, and League of Women Voters were all pro-reform activists. Drs. Taussig and Kelsey and Eleanor Roosevelt in particular all helped in a layering process whereby women's health and safety were brought front and center to the FDA's attention, based on the sulfanilamide and thalidomide disasters. The historical institutionalist process of layering combined with discursive institutionalism as in Carpenter's three-faces-of-power analysis (decision-making, nondecisions, and reputation) saw Congress legislate more power to the FDA over time. These powers included pharma's requirement to prove safety (1938), efficacy (1962), and other changes, including the rise of the prescription and generics industries.

The theories of Baumgartner and Jones on policy punctuations, as adapted by Ceccoli to the FDA, can be combined with Carpenter's institutionalist history of the FDA. While Carpenter rejects the abrupt policy punctuations of the Baumgartner and Jones model as too drastic, his three-faces-of-power framework, concerning decisions, nondecisions, and organizational reputation, is helpful for this feminist institutionalist analysis of the FDA and the U.S. pharma policymaking system. From Baumgartner and Jones and thus Ceccoli, this study describes two U.S. policy punctuations on women's reproductive drugs. The first was during a period when women were not very well descriptively represented and the substantive representation of them concerning contraception's availability and funding was done through presidents concerned with global population growth. Still, that framework proved a durable one to help women until social conservative politicians elected after 1980 started rolling the framework back. The second policy punctuation has been largely unfriendly to women's reproductive drug policy, as evidenced by the Republican-based conversions to previously embedded national structures.

In his description of the continuity of FDA decision-making criteria over time, including criteria not yet formally encoded in the laws, Carpenter provides a thorough analysis of why punctuated equilibria alone do not explain the FDA's history. Historical continuity including the layering model enables a description, like Streeck and Thelen's, as to when certain parts of institutions or a political system change at differential rates. Attentiveness to continuity also enables feminist institutionalists to understand the ability of certain rules to persist in the separation of powers systems, whereby in majority parliamentarian systems, they could be done away with completely. Thus, for example, the Obama administration has kept the White House faith-based office, and Congress and the president have kept abstinence-based funding in the budget.

NOTES

1. Daniel Carpenter, *Reputation and Power: Organizational Image and Pharmaceutical Regulation at the FDA* (Princeton, NJ: Princeton University Press, 2010).

2. Karen O'Connor and Larry Sabato, *American Government: Continuity and Change* (New York: Pearson Education Inc., 2008), 328–30.

3. Theodore J. Lowi, *The End of Liberalism: Ideology, Policy, and the Crisis of Authority* (New York: Norton, 1969).

4. Sidney Tarrow, *Power in Movement: Social Movements and Contentious Politics* (Cambridge: Cambridge University Press, 1998).

5. Peter Bachrach and Morton S. Baratz, "The Two Faces of Power," *American Political Science Review* 56, no. 4 (December 1962): 947–52.

6. Barbara Sinclair, *Unorthodox Lawmaking: New Legislative Processes in the U.S. Congress*, 3rd ed. (Washington, DC: Congressional Quarterly, Inc., 2007), 65, 100–101.

7. "History of the FDA: Commissioners and Deputy Commissioners," *U.S. Food and Drug Administration*, www.fda.gov.

8. Theodore J. Lowi, *The End of Liberalism: Ideology, Policy, and the Crisis of Authority* (New York: Norton, 1969); Sidney Tarrow, *Power in Movement: Social Movements and Contentious Politics* (Cambridge: Cambridge University Press, 1998); and Walter Dean Burnham, *Critical Elections: And the Mainsprings of American Politics* (New York: W. W. Norton and Company, 1971).

9. Frank Baumgartner and Bryan Jones, *Agendas and Instability in American Politics* (Chicago, IL: University of Chicago Press, 1993); Frank Baumgartner and Bryan Jones, eds., *Policy Dynamics* (Chicago, IL: University of Chicago Press, 2002); and John Kingdon, *Agendas, Alternatives and Public Policies*, 2nd ed. (London: Longman and Pearson, 1984).

10. Carpenter, *Reputation and Power,* Introduction and 73–228.

11. Ibid., 120.

12. The cases include *Griswold v. CT,* 381 US 479 (1965); *Eisenstadt v. Baird,* 405 US 438 (1972); and *Roe v. Wade,* 410 US 113 (1973).

13. Mary Brown Bullock, *The Oil Prince's Legacy: Rockefeller Philanthropy in China* (Palo Alto, CA: Stanford University Press, 2011) and Ansley J. Coale, *Rapid Population Change in China, 1952–1982* (Washington, DC: National Academies Press, June 1984).

14. *Webster v. Reproductive Health Services,* 492 US 490 (1989) and *Casey v. Pennsylvania,* 505 US 833 (1992).

15. See Wolfgang Streeck and Kathleen Thelen, "Introduction," in *Beyond Continuity: Institutional Change in Advanced Political Economies,* eds. Wolfgang Streeck and Kathleen Thelen (Oxford: Oxford University Press, 2005), 22–26 and Jacob Hacker, "Policy Drift: The Hidden Politics of US Welfare State Retrenchment," in Streck and Thelen, *Beyond Continuity,* 40–82.

16. Carpenter, *Reputation and Power,* 637–38.

17. David J. Ravenscraft and William F. Long, "Paths to Creating Value in Pharmaceutical Mergers," in *Mergers and Productivity,* ed. Steven N. Kaplan (Chicago, IL: University of Chicago Press, 2000), 294–95, http://www.nber.org/chapters/c8653.pdf.

18. "Import Program Overview," *US Food and Drug Administration,* http://www.fda.gov/ForIndustry/ImportProgram/ImportProgramOverview/default.htm.

19. Denise Chicoine, "RU-486 in the US and Great Britain: A Case Study in Gender Bias," *Boston College International and Comparative Law Review* 16, no. 1 (December 1993): 87.

20. Carpenter, *Reputation and Power.*

21. "The Fortune 500," *CNNMoney,* http://money.cnn.com/magazines/fortune/fortune500/2011/index.html.

22. Marcia Angell, "Over and Above: Excess in the Pharmaceutical Industry," *Canadian Medical Association Journal* 171, no. 12 (2004): 1451–53, http://www.cmaj.ca/content/171/12/1451.full.

23. Stephen Ceccoli, *Pill Politics: Drugs and the FDA* (Boulder, CO: Lynne Rienner Publishers, 2004), 55.

24. Henry Grabowski and John Vernon, *The Regulation of Pharmaceuticals* (Washington, DC: American Enterprise Institute, 1983) and Ceccoli, *Pill Politics.*

25. Ceccoli, *Pill Politics,* 59.

26. "History," US Food and Drug Administration, www.fda.gov.

27. Wallace Jannsen, "The Story of the Laws behind the Labels," *FDA Consumer* 15, no. 5 (June 1981): 32, cited in Ceccoli, *Pill Politics,* 59.

28. Ceccoli, *Pill Politics,* 59.

29. A. Hunter Dupree, *Science in the Federal Government: A History of Policy and Activities to 1940* (Cambridge, MA: Harvard University Press, 1957), 176 and Jannsen, "The Story of the Laws," 32, cited in Ceccoli, *Pill Politics,* 59.

30. Ceccoli, *Pill Politics,* 60–65.

31. Ibid., 60.

32. See Doug McAdam, John McCarthy, and Mayer Zald, *Comparative Perspectives on Social Movements: Political Opportunities, Mobilizing Structures and Cultural Framings* (Cambridge: Cambridge University Press, 1996).

33. Peter Temin, *Taking Your Medicine: Drug Regulation in the United States* (Cambridge, MA: Harvard University Press, 1980), 27, cited in Ceccoli, *Pill Politics*, 60.

34. Ceccoli, *Pill Politics*, 61–62.

35. Marc Eisner, *Regulatory Politics in Transition*, 2nd ed. (Baltimore, MD: Johns Hopkins University Press, 2000).

36. Peter Temin, *Taking Your Medicine*, 32, cited in Ceccoli, *Pill Politics*, 63.

37. Barbara Martin, M.D., "Elixir Sulfanilamide Tragedy Calls for Improved Legislation," *Pathophilia*, March 13, 2009, http://bmartinmd.com/cgi-bin/mt/mt-search.cgi?search=Elixir+Sulfanilamide+Tragedy+Calls+for+Improved+Legislation&IncludeBlogs=1 and Donna Young, "Documentary Examines Sulfanilamide Deaths of 1937," *American Society of Health-System Pharmacists*, December 5, 2003, http://www.ashp.org/menu/News/PharmacyNews/NewsArticle.aspx?id=1443.

38. Ceccoli, *Pill Politics*, 68–69.

39. Charles Jackson, *Food and Drug Legislation in the New Deal* (Princeton, NJ: Princeton University Press, 1970), 29.

40. "Sulfanilamide Elixir Deaths Bring Demand for US Curb," *St. Louis Post-Dispatch*, November 2, 1937 and Dutcher, R., "Sulfanilamide Elixir Deaths," *Anniston Star*, November 7, 1937, 4, both cited in Martin, "Elixir Sulfanilamide Tragedy."

41. Young, "Documentary Examines Sulfanilamide Deaths."

42. Carpenter, *Reputation and Power*, 107.

43. Ibid., 110–11.

44. Ibid., 100–106.

45. Ibid., 254, 258.

46. Ceccoli, *Pill Politics*, 70–71.

47. Carpenter, *Reputation and Power*, 100–18.

48. Ibid., 100.

49. Ibid., 103–106.

50. Ibid., 637–38.

51. Walter Armstrong, "The FDA's Approvable Problem," *PharmExec*, November 1, 2007, http://www.pharmexec.com/pharmexec/article/articleDetail.jsp?id=469652.

52. "Changing the Face of Medicine, Biography: Dr. Frances Kathleen Oldham Kelsey," *National Library of Medicine*, http://www.nlm.nih.gov/changingthefaceofmedicine/physicians/biography_182.html.

53. Frances Kelsey, "Denial of Approval for Thalidomide in the United States" (Speech, National Library of Medicine, Bethesda, MD, December 9, 1993).

54. Ibid.

55. London Sunday Times, *Suffer the Children: The Story of Thalidomide* (New York: Viking Press, 1979), cited in George J. Annas, M.D., and Sherman Elias, M.D., "Thalido-

mide and the *Titanic:* Reconstructing the Technology Tragedies of the Twentieth Century," *American Journal of Public Health* 89, no. 1 (January 1999): 98–101.

56. Sheryl Gay Stolberg, "37 Years Later, a Second Chance for Thalidomide," *New York Times,* September 23, 1997, http://www.nytimes.com/1997/09/23/us/37-years-later-a-second-chance-for-thalidomide.html?pagewanted=all&src=pm.

57. "Changing the Face of Medicine: Dr. Frances Kathleen Oldham Kelsey" and "Changing the Face of Medicine: Dr. Helen Brooke Taussig," *National Library of Medicine,* http://www.nlm.nih.gov/changingthefaceofmedicine/physicians/.

58. Carpenter, *Reputation and Power,* 232.

59. Ibid., 234.

60. Ibid., 235.

61. Ibid., 236.

62. Ibid., 238.

63. Ibid., 238–69.

64. "Medicine: Sleeping Pill Nightmare," *Time,* February 23, 1962, http://www.time.com/time/magazine/article/0,9171,895929,00.html and Lisa A. Seidman and Noreen Warren, "Pharmaceutical Regulation in the US: History and a Case Study," *Bio-Link,* June 2001, http://www.bio-link.org/GMP/KELPOST.html.

65. Seidman and Warren, "Pharmaceutical Regulation in the US."

66. Kathleen L. Neeley, "Kelsey, Frances Kathleen Oldham," *Chemistry: Foundations and Applications,* January 2004, http://www.encyclopedia.com/doc/1G2-3400900275.html.

67. Scott P. Glauberman, "The Real Thalidomide Baby: The Evolution of the FDA in the Shadow of Thalidomide, 1960–1997," *Food and Drug Law* (Winter 1997), http://leda.law.harvard.edu/leda/data/389/.

68. Carpenter, *Reputation and Power,* 237, 270.

69. Ibid., 269.

70. Elizabeth Siegel Watkins, *On the Pill: A Social History of Oral Contraceptives, 1950–1970* (Baltimore, MD: The Johns Hopkins University Press, 1998), 120.

71. Ibid.

72. Ibid.

73. Martha Rumore, Pharm.D., J.D., F.A.Ph.A., "The Hatch-Waxman Act—25 Years Later: Keeping the Pharmaceutical Scales Balanced," *Pharmacy Times,* August 15, 2009, http://www.pharmacytimes.com/publications/supplement/2009/genericsupplement0809/generic-hatchwaxman-0809.

74. Ibid.

75. Hasneen Karbalai, "The Hatch-Waxman (Im) Balancing Act," *LEDA at Harvard School,* 1–2, http://leda.law. harvard.edu/leda/data/551/Paper1.html.

76. Rumore, "The Hatch-Waxman Act."

77. Ceccoli, *Pill Politics,* 105–106.

78. Steven Epstein, *Impure Science: AIDS, Activism and the Politics of Knowledge* (Berkeley, CA: University of California Press, 1996), 8, cited in Ceccoli, *Pill Politics,* 106.

79. Ibid.

80. Ibid.

81. C. F. Larry Heimann, *Acceptable Risks: Politics, Policy, and Risky Technologies* (Ann Arbor, MI: University of Michigan Press, 1997), cited in Ceccoli, *Pill Politics*, 104.

82. David Kessler, *A Question of Intent* (New York: Public Affairs Press, 2001), 403, cited in Ceccoli, *Pill Politics*, 104.

83. Ibid.

84. Ibid. and Sean Hennessy, Pharm.D., and Brian L. Strom, M.D., "PDUFA Reauthorization-Drug Safety's Golden Moment of Opportunity?" *New England Journal of Medicine* 356, no. 17 (April 26, 2007): 1703–4, http://www.nejm.org/doi/full/10.1056/NEJMp078048.

85. Ibid.

86. "NEJM: User-Fee Law Makes the FDA Accountable to Big Pharma," *NewsInferno*, May 3, 2007, http://www.newsinferno.com/legal-news/nejm-user-fee-law-makes-fda-%E2%80%9Caccountable%E2%80%9D-to-big-pharma/1558.

87. Watkins, 139–40.

88. Ilyssa Hollander, "Viagra's Rise above Women's Health Issues: An Analysis of the Social and Political Influences on Drug Approvals in the US and Japan," *Social Sciences and Medicine* 62 (2006): 683–93, http://www.ssds.net/ssds-products/peer-reviewed-pubs/Hollander--Viagra.pdf.

3

The Development of the Pill

The birth-control pill is the first of this book's four case studies of pharmaceuticals related to women's reproductive systems. This chapter's argument is that the public discourse around women's proper situation of not having reproductive autonomy has been successfully used twice in the U.S. history to deny women the ability to control their fertility. The manipulation of political discourse is best explained by the model of discursive institutionalism, in which first the Comstock coalition from 1873 to 1915 and then the Vatican and New Right since 1980 have lobbied the U.S. state to achieve their ends at the expense of women.[1]

In the social conservative view, access to information about contraception and abortion is inherently corrupting women's and children's morals and a blow to a theoretical construction of manhood.[2] The role of discursive power as wielded by contraception and abortion opponents has been to provide cover for U.S. pharma. In the first three case studies considered in this book, U.S. pharma, a huge and highly profitable set of corporations with a global reach, consistently claimed women's reproductive drugs were too risky to develop, because it would put them in the path of social conservative boycotts. In the fourth case study on Gardasil, risks to women were mostly ignored by social conservatives in the rush to give Merck a blockbuster drug to replace Vioxx in 2006.

In Comstock's time, the central nexus of political power in which he operated to become the main actor prosecuting Americans on loosely defined obscenity issues included Congress, successive presidents and postmasters general, the U.S. Postal Service, and state legislators.[3] This particular chapter's discussion covers primarily the run-up to the first policy period on women's reproductive rights, ending in the early 1960s when the Pill was approved by the Food and Drug Administration (FDA). While women were not represented in great numbers in state institutions from 1960 to 1980, that was the period of greatest expansion of women's contraceptive and abortion rights. A chief reason for that was the interest of Presidents Johnson and Nixon in furthering U.S. agricultural industries, of which contraception was a part, and addressing the global population issue. Public funding was available in the most comprehensive format for contraception and abortion under the Johnson, Nixon, and Ford presidencies.

Other relevant pieces from institutionalist and other political theories for this chapter include the following. The historical institutionalist models of layering and conversion are applicable. The primary examples of layering in the years up to the 1960s included pharma's adoption of anti-choice themes to deny contraceptive development, but there was a positive example as well. The positive example was found in Margaret Sanger and Katherine McCormick's advocacy of the Pill. Sanger's work from the turn of the 20th century until the early 1960s not only helped layer a pro-contraception standpoint into the pharma industry, but it also brought about a conversion of the private–public sector institutions on reproductive policymaking for a short time. In that conversion, lasting into the mid-1970s, companies realized that contraception could be profitable, particularly when publicly-funded. Another important element of that conversion was that from 1960 until *Roe v. Wade* in 1973, the U.S. Catholic Church was generally not a vocal anti-contraception lobbyist.[4] In addition, Lowi's iron-triangle theory regarding the continued domination of the U.S. pharma policymaking by a trio of male-dominated institutions until 1960 is demonstrated.

OVERVIEW OF RELATED U.S. OBSCENITY, IMPORT, AND TARIFF LAWS

The United States has been subject to Comstock-style prohibitions concerning obscenity, the government's power to define it, and associated restrictions on women's access to reproductive information, contraception, and abortion for the majority of its history. Indeed, the Comstock Act's provision against abortion advertising is still contained in the federal criminal code. Congress removed the anti-contraception language in 1971. Interestingly, the cause of Congressional action in 1971 was that Representative James Scheuer of New York had been working on the issue since 1967, when a constituent was made to throw her diaphragm into New York Harbor on reentry into the United States.[5] Scheuer was a liberal Democratic 13-term U.S. House member, and a contraceptive supporter.[6] As noted by then U.S. Representative to the United Nations George H. W. Bush in a Foreword to a book by Johns Hopkins Public Health Professor Phyllis Piotrow, Scheuer was part of a bipartisan coalition supporting birth control, other members "including Senator Ernest Gruening (R-AK), Representative Bob Taft (R-OH), Representative and then Senator Bill Fulbright (D-AR), Senator Joe Tydings (D-MD), Senator Bob Packwood (R-OR), Senator Alan Cranston (D-CA), and many others from both parties and every section of the country."[7] At that time, Bush was very open about being pro-contraception, a stance that was politically possible for Republicans before 1980.

A majority of the states had prohibitions against obscenity in the early 19th century. Anthony Comstock, a puritanical Congregationalist activist from New York, who had amassed funding from the founders of the Young Men's Christian Association, had sufficient power through his state-based organization to persuade Congress to pass the federal Comstock Act in 1873. Twenty-four states also passed Comstock prohibitions, specifically containing anti-contraception and anti-abortion language.[8] As noted by Lori Maurice, the first federal law regarding obscenity and the mails was on the books by 1865. Under the Comstock Act, "the obscenity law was amended to provide that the term 'indecent' shall include matter tending to arson, murder, or assassination." The "publication, distribution, and possession of information about or devices or medications for 'unlawful' abortion or contraception" were criminalized under this act.[9]

The Comstock Act was passed at the end of the Grant administration, and dealt only with domestically produced obscenity. Similar to the ways in which many anti-reproductive choice amendments have been passed in Congress in recent years, through supplemental budget reconciliation bills once the fiscal year has passed, the Comstock legislation was rushed through Congress in a special procedure of its own, notes Maurice.[10] From 1873 until his death in 1915, Comstock was appointed a special agent of the U.S. Postal Service, with the unilateral power to determine the extent of obscenity and to apprehend those purportedly practicing it. Comstock used this power to define obscenity very broadly, and did not restrict himself to postal matters.[11] By the end of his life, Comstock boasted of having arrested more than 3,600 people.

Comstock's zealous pursuit of the Sangers resulted in many court cases, the first of which watered down the Comstock language, but not its enforcement. When Sanger appealed a 1918 conviction, the state appeals court held that "contraceptive devices could legally be promoted for the cure and prevention of disease."[12] However, it was not until the *One Package* decision of 1936 that contraceptive devices could specifically be imported by licensed physicians for clients' use that a viable defense for physicians was established.[13]

In the U.S. separation of powers system, social movement entrepreneurs often turn to the courts when legislation or legislators prove to be unhelpful. It was Margaret Sanger's goal since the late 19th century to overturn anti-contraception laws and so she and her colleagues often bounced back and forth, and to state legislatures, in pursuit of their beliefs. What is also interesting and is shown throughout the book is that reproductive choice opponents in Congress could often thwart women's access to contraceptives or information about them through various tariff and import acts.

The legal fiction of regulation as being beneficial to all was shown by the Imported Drugs Act of 1848. Ceccoli notes that it was intended to "stop the entry of adulterated drugs from overseas." As evidence, he cites one of the official FDA historians' statements that "the US had become the world's dumping ground for counterfeit, contaminated, diluted and decomposed drug materials."[14] Of course, the goal of keeping harmful drugs out of the country is a good one. The problem arises when customs and agriculture inspectors are given broad powers, as they usually are, to determine which goods are admissible. Unfortunately for women, this exercise of state power often meant denial of their access to a variety of contraceptives.

In 1930, Congress passed the Smoot-Hawley Act, sponsored by two western members, Senator Smoot of Utah and Representative Hawley of Oregon. The aim of the legislation was a misguided belief that levying large tariffs on imported goods would bolster the U.S. industry. The law helped usher in the Depression, not least due to protectionist tariffs then imposed by trade partners. By 1932, "US exports and imports had plunged by nearly 70 percent."[15]

Perhaps unsurprisingly, tariff bills, like Congressional budgets, can have moralistic policies embedded in them. Probably unfortunately, Margaret Sanger tipped her hand in this scenario. Legislative targeting from the 1920s onward was part of Phase II of Sanger's activist career as described in one of the last parts of the chapter. Sanger had been lobbying Congress for a vehicle by which to undo the Comstock prohibitions on domestic and imported contraception and abortion materials. She had various allies, none of whom had much power, introduce bills for her to this effect.[16]

Part of the answer is to be found in *Time*'s description of the American Medical Association's (AMA's) annual conference in New Orleans in 1932. The then House member (later Speaker) John McCormack—a member of the Knights of Columbus and Hibernian Society, both organizations strongly represented among Irish Catholics in Massachusetts—played legislative games with the bill.

Part of the account comes from the AMA *Journal* of 1932, which described "Mrs. Sanger as having been in an exasperated fix."[17]

The key piece of this puzzle is that the end product of the Smoot-Hawley Act was not just conservatism in trade, but also in morality. Senator Smoot (R-UT), "a senior member of the Church of the Latter-Day Saints of Jesus Christ" (Mormon) and chair of the Senate Finance Committee, inserted Section 305 as an amendment to the Smoot-Hawley Tariff. Section 305 restated the Comstock Act verbatim with the exception of having the "importation of obscene pictures" removed. Since the bill was tariff legislation, the House Chair of Ways and Means (conveniently the bill's cosponsor Representative Hawley) and Senator Smoot were able to accomplish all the stickhandling. Addition of Section 305 into Smoot-Hawley gave the Comstock provisions even more of a broad international sweep than they previously enjoyed.[18]

Sanger's response was to stage an event of public theater to test the scope of the law. She had amassed a collection of contraceptive-related items seized by customs officials over the years, which had been intended for physicians. Sanger and her colleague at the American Birth Control League, Dr. Hannah Stone, arranged with Japanese contacts to have 120 diaphragms sent to Dr. Stone for use in her private practice. To make sure that the event went off as per Sanger's wishes, customs officials were informed of this transaction in advance.[19] Unsurprisingly, the diaphragms were seized by the U.S. Customs.

In response, Sanger and Dr. Stone filed suit first in the federal district court of Southern New York in 1934, and it took two years for their case to be heard. However, the end result was helpful because in January 1936, District Court Judge Grover Moscowitz held that Dr. Stone could legally receive contraceptive devices sent by Japanese physicians. Another important part of the decision was that Section 305 of the Smoot-Hawley Act did not cover contraceptives dispensed by physicians. Some have stated that the public opinion of birth control at the time was 71 percent in favor and that may have helped the judge reach his decision. In a similar vein, Reed has noted that by the 1930s, with or without a dispensary license, "birth control clinics in the US were doing a booming business."[20] On the other hand, it would be wise to recall the 1932 *Time* article about the AMA Conference before reaching a universalistic conclusion. While FDR's solicitor general was instructed to appeal the decision, Sanger and Stone prevailed in the federal appellate court as well. In that decision of December 1936, Judge Augustus Hand wrote that Section 305 of the Smoot-Hawley Act had joined the word "unlawful" with abortion, but not with contraception, thus allowing importation of contraceptives for medical use. In 1937, the AMA voted to start supporting birth control as a public policy.

THE FINANCIAL INTEREST OF THE PHARMA INDUSTRY

On one hand, the U.S. pharma industry claimed from the 1940s onward that it was not interested in funding research into finding alternatives to animal-based cholesterol, and specifically that it was not interested in funding research on hormonal contraception. Even by the 1930s, however, while still mainly illegal and usually unsafe compounds, contraceptives brought in 250 million dollars annually.[21] Particularly since the second half of the 20th century, pharma companies make decisions on which drugs to promote for FDA approval based on their blockbuster potential. Since blockbuster drugs are the lifeblood of the pharma industry, the FDA is usually supportive of their development. Blockbusters are defined as yielding a minimum of 1 billion dollars annually.[22]

The House Commerce and Energy Committee, charged with overseeing the FDA, is the oldest House standing committee. Similarly, the FDA is one of the oldest federal agencies. The ties between pharma and government (executive and legislative) have had a long time to solidify, one of the still-existing examples of Lowi's famous iron-triangle formulation regarding the Department of Agriculture.[23] The two public-sector points of the triangle are the House Energy and Commerce Committee (legislative branch) and the FDA (executive branch), and the private-sector point is the pharma lobby. As of 2010, the Pharmaceutical Researchers and Manufacturers of America (the lobby known as PhRMA) was fourth in the list of contributors to federal campaigns.[24] The head of PhRMA at the time was former Congressman Billy Tauzin, also former chair of the House Commerce and Energy Committee.

As studies by Dr. Marcia Angell and journalist Fran Hawthorne have shown, drug companies do not foot most of the bill for pharma research in the United States. Instead, the federal government—typically through the Department of Health and Human Services and its units the National Institutes of Health, Centers for Disease Control, and National Cancer Institute (NCI)—is the largest funder. Universities receive and partner with the government funds to provide more money and research labs, and sometimes state governments help fund research. Therefore, many of the companies' protestations about funding research are even less believable. As stated by Philip Hilts, "today there are 10,000 to 15,000 drugs on the market, and the World Health Organization considers that a properly-equipped pharmacy needs only 350 of them." He has also noted that "ninety-five percent of the new drugs put on the market are 'me too' drugs . . . almost identical to a half dozen already on the market."[25] In other words, the U.S. pharma industry has pushed most of the risk-taking (financial and otherwise) onto its researchers and the government that funds them, yet is able to reap fantastic rewards. As noted by Senator Bernie Sanders of Vermont:

Even the New York Yankees sometimes lose. . . . But one organization never loses, and that organization has hundreds of victories to its credit and zero defeats in the United States Congress. And that is the pharmaceutical industry.[26]

CHEMICAL RESEARCH AND DEVELOPMENT LEADING TO THE BIRTH-CONTROL PILL

The research and development on steroid hormones began in the late 19th century in Europe. Since the raw material needed was cholesterol, scientists obtained it from animals and humans. Scientists soon learned the potential for regulating women's menstrual cycles and fertility. Since research for the Pill formed the largest quest to regulate women's hormones, it formed the basis for research on other reproductive drugs, such as the morning-after pill, IUD, and RU-486.

At the heart of the hormonal research conducted since the 19th century are the following facts. The types of contraceptive pills eventually approved for marketing from 1960 onward contained a combination of synthetic progesterone (progestins) and synthetic estrogens (sometimes called estrols). All hormones are classified as either steroid hormones, or protein (peptide) hormones. Steroid hormones are based on the sterol substance cholesterol, which can be of plant or animal origin. These hormones are secreted and synthesized by the placenta or endocrine glands including ovaries or testes and the adrenal cortex. All steroid hormones contain the steroid nucleus and three six-member rings, a five-member ring, and a unique side chain. While steroids are a "fat-soluble organic compound," hormones are the "chemical messenger produced by the endocrine glands."[27] There are five types of steroid hormones, including androgens and estrogens that are related to sexual differentiation and function. Third, progestins regulate the menstrual cycle and pregnancy. Fourth, mineralocorticoids mainly regulate the excretion of salt and water by the kidneys. Fifth, glucocorticoids affect carbohydrate, lipid, and protein metabolism and are involved in inflammatory and stress reactions. On the other hand, protein or peptide hormones (nonsteroidal) are derived from long chains of amino acids.[28]

Due to the inconsistent nature of government and private-sector supports for hormonal research, parallel research endeavors developed in the world. In the 20th century, scientists learned to extract cholesterol from plant sources in addition to the other origins. One could draw lines across the globe to demonstrate the research connections from the late 19th to about the mid-20th centuries. Such a global map of research and knowledge connections would often involve U.S. or European scientists, with U.S. scientists often going to Europe to pursue research illegal at home, as happened under the Comstock Act of 1873.

However, when the climate for hormonal research tightened in both Europe and the United States following major losses of life in World War I, scientists had to do much of their research underground. Historically, until about the 1950s, the knowledge transfer in pharma research, including on reproductive drugs, was an arrow flowing from Europe to the United States. Much of the U.S. pharma industry was developed by seizing the U.S.-based assets of foreign-owned companies, a wartime practice.[29]

Starting around 1940, the global map of knowledge and research links included Mexico, which became a large source of and willing partner in providing raw plant materials as a better source of cholesterol from which to synthesize hormones. Of course, it should also be added that while scientists and researchers were often willing to collaborate, of necessity, governments and pharma companies wished to maintain a strictly competitive relationship. Tariffs on raw and finished materials, customs inspections, and import quotas, not to mention denying research funding, are all ways in which governments can tilt the balance in favor of one at the expense of another.

The Austro-Hungarian area led the world in creating steroid hormones in the early 19th century. In 1921, Dr. Ludwig Haberlandt, an Austrian researcher, claimed that he had created a steroid hormone.[30] Hormone-based research had occurred in Europe since the 1880s. In the 1920s, sex hormones "began to be used in Europe to treat gynaecological disorders, such as menstrual irregularity, infertility and menopausal complaints."[31] The same did not occur in the United States until 1957. By the early 20th century, Europeans had access to a number of organotherapies (derived from animal organs in slaughterhouses) that were unregulated, were available without a prescription, and sold for a profit from druggists. Also, from the late 19th until the early 20th centuries, scientists in the United States and mainly Europe were successfully isolating hormones that would prevent ovulation, including estrogen from animals' ovaries and progesterone from the corpus luteum, or ruptured egg sacs.[32] By the end of the 1920s, Dr. Haberlandt began to make overtures to German companies Farben and Merck to "produce a progesterone-based hormonal contraceptive."[33] Neither company was willing to engage in the perceived risk, although in 1928, Haberlandt did secure a contract with the Hungarian company Gedeon Richter (by then a leader in hormonal research) to produce his contraceptive discovery. By 1930, Richter had commercially registered a compound based on Haberlandt's research, called Infecundin.

As a clinician but not a physician, Haberlandt faced the same issue encountered 25 years later by Dr. Gregory Pincus, also a clinician who helped develop the U.S. pill. Clinicians were not allowed to perform human studies. Haberlandt was denied promotion at his university, and Pincus was denied tenure at

Harvard, based on claims that their research was risky and out of the academic mainstream.

Haberlandt died in 1932, but Infecundin received human trials at a women's hospital in Innsbruck, Switzerland in 1934. While the study's results were never published, Richter successfully renewed its license on the product through the 1940s. There were rumors of a related compound called Profecundin tested in Nazi Germany. Gedeon Richter always denied having marketed Infecundin in Hungary as a contraceptive during the 1930s and 1940s. It only officially began marketing the product in Hungary in 1966, six years after Searle had taken the heat as the first producer of a contraceptive pill, Enovid.[34]

U.S. scientists mainly had to perform reproductive-related research on the Q.T. until the 1960s. Even though U.S. researchers could not be open about their animal-based research as could their European counterparts, an American scientist, George Corner was the first in the 1920s to establish that a woman's menstrual cycle released different types of hormones at different points, with a high load of estrogen in the first half and then progesterone that ended a woman's menstrual period.[35] Corner's research findings confirmed those of Professor Fuller Albright of Harvard University, who in the late 1930s and 1940s "argued that fertility could be controlled by a combination of estrogen and progesterone." His suggested medications were a combination of stilboestrol and progesterone, "remarkably similar to the one later used in developing the first marketable pill."[36]

As Marks discusses, synthetic, nonsteroidal estrogen (called stilboestrol in the United Kingdom, where it was first processed, and diethylstilboestrol in the United States) had been developed by an eminent British biochemist, Sir Charles Dodds, by the 1930s. Dodds had been funded by the British Medical Research Council, but reflecting the ambivalence present in the 1930s, the Council was "less than enthusiastic about its use as a contraceptive." Part of the reason for the lukewarm reception of the scientific breakthrough was that, as with emergency contraception nearly a century later, it worked mainly by preventing implantation of a fertilized egg.[37] In the 1930s, the British government officially framed the prevention of implantation as causing an abortion, and thus placed stilboestrol on its official list of poisons in 1939. However, by the 1940s, stilboestrol was widely prescribed in the United States and the Netherlands for the prevention of miscarriage and was being fed to farm animals.

Given that the 1930s climate on animal-based hormonal contraceptive research was not openly supportive, many leading scientists began to turn to plant-based derivatives for their initial material. In the 1930s, chemist Russell Marker of Pennsylvania State University, a leading researcher in distilling chemical substances from complex organic materials, was looking for a plant-based cholesterol substance. The Japanese had isolated such a substance in 1936 from a plant known as *Dioscorea tokoro*.[38] A related event spurring U.S. researchers to look to plants for cholesterol sources was that five major European companies—the Swiss CIBA, the German Boehringer, the Dutch Organon, and the French Roussel—drew up a "joint agreement in 1937 which allowed them to deploy each others' inventions."[39] This action formed a monopolistic agreement, designed to keep the European companies ahead of the U.S.-based ones in the area of steroidal hormone research.

At the time, Parke-Davis was the only producer of steroid hormones in the United States, specifically the female hormone oestrone. Eager to retain its lead position in the steroid market, yet not wishing to publicly be identified with contraceptive research, Parke-Davis was willing to fund Marker in his research for plants that would yield the highest level of cholesterol (sapogenin). As with mammalian sources of cholesterol, vast quantities were needed to synthesize hormones. Marker was able to produce synthetic progesterone (progestin) from the sarsaparilla plant. By 1940, "he had developed a five-stage chemical process for the conversion of sapogenins (from sarsaparilla) into progesterone, which taken three stages further, produced the male hormone testosterone."[40] Testosterone was vital to sex-hormone research because it could "be manipulated to make analogues of female hormones."[41] The sarsaparilla-based process was deemed too expensive by Parke-Davis. Since other sources of sapogenins, such as soya were becoming available in the United States, Parke-Davis opted out of funding Marker's further travels.[42]

Marker decided to pursue research in the Southwest United States and in Mexico. In this, he was on his own, funding his own travels and research. In Mexico, in 1940, Marker found a plant that was a rich source of sapogenins, the *cabeza de negro*, a wild yam. He had to set up a laboratory to produce the progesterone, and fund the whole enterprise. Given that "most Mexican chemists at the time worked either in the petroleum or sugar industry," Marker had to turn to scientists trained mainly in Europe to work in his Mexican-based lab. The Mexican environment was more loosely regulated at the time than the United States regarding research subjects.

Marker had been employing a very rudimentary operation in which the dried *Cabeza de negro* was brought to Mexico City for further processing to extract the plant-based steroid compounds, sapogenins, including diosgenin. These extracts were turned into a syrup, which Marker then brought to the United States and, borrowing a friend's laboratory, turned into synthesized progesterone.

By 1944, Marker had formed a new company, Syntex, which soon led the field in international supplies of progesterone.[43] Marker soon left the company over a payment dispute, taking his notebooks with him. He formed a new company,

Diosynth in 1949, based on his research with a root related to the *Cabeza* plant, the *Barbasco* plant, and the Dioscorea plant.[44]

Other European-born scientists, including Professors George Rosenkrantz, Carl Djerassi, and Alexander Zaffaroni, were hired to replace Marker at Syntex.[45] These men had much experience in Europe producing synthesized hormones for research, and Djerassi had previously worked for CIBA, the Swiss company that held the patent for cholesterol. Djerassi was "encouraged by Syntex as part of its drive to fulfill its industrial potential and expand its range of steroidal intermediaries."[46] A brilliant Mexican graduate student, Luis Miramontes, was recruited from UNAM (the National Autonomous University of Mexico) to work with Djerassi, and is the one credited with performing the synthesis of a progestin and estrogen–based product, called norethisterone. Marks characterizes this substance as the "first compound capable of being used as an oral contraceptive." Norethisterone is also referred to as norethindrone. On one hand, the synthetic progesterone was much less expensive than its natural counterpart, yet on the other, it had to be used in high quantities, which produced unacceptable side effects in trial subjects.[47] Carl Djerassi announced the success of "synthesizing orally active analogues of progesterone" at a meeting of the American Chemical Society in 1952. The compound he formulated was named 19-nor progestin, since "at the number 19 position in the progesterone molecule, it lacked a side chain of one carbon and three hydrogen atoms (a 'methyl group')."[48]

Marks cites Djerassi's 1992 book, *The Pill, Pygmy Chimps and I* to the effect that Miramontes and Djerassi, while understanding that their production of norethisterone could work "for problems such as menstrual disorders and recurrent miscarriage," did not appreciate the contraceptive potential of the synthesized compound.[49] This interpretation strains credulity, since probably every chemist working with hormones since at least the 1920s had understood that there was a potential contraceptive impact involved, and companies including Parke-Davis, Merck, Searle, and Gedeon Richter refused to fund them on one of two grounds. The first was that the research would only affect a few women and thus was not going to be cost-effective, or that the potential for contraceptive use violated the U.S. law at the time. Marks reports that scientist Dr. Roy Hertz at the NCI in Bethesda, Maryland, was "one of the first to expound on norethisterone's contraceptive potential." Since the 1930s, Hertz had been involved with the previous research on progestational compounds. The results showed that when taken orally, the synthetic norethisterone "was much more potent than pure progesterone taken either orally or injected."[50] At the time, it was clear at least that many reproductive problems (such as miscarriage and menstrual pain) could be treated from these drugs.

Various U.S. companies, including Searle, Upjohn, and Merck, were involved in the "race to duplicate and improve on Marker's processes for corticosteroid development," leading to the creation of many compounds from Marker's molecule.[51] Companies were happy to benefit from the research that Marker did on his own and with colleagues in Mexico. There were still problems in getting the raw materials from which to synthesize the steroid hormones. In 1951, Syntex convinced the Mexican agriculture minister to grant it the sole license for the collection of the *Barbasco* and wild yam (*Cabeza de Negro*) roots in the forests. Even more powerful was President Aleman's mandate that followed it, imposing a tax on the exportation of the roots and related intermediate compounds. Syntex was the only company with the knowledge to process intermediates not subject to the export tax.[52]

Other companies started to oppose Syntex's monopolistic practices. During World War II, U.S. companies were significantly helped along by the nationalist expropriation of German-held Schering Corporation patents for steroid manufacture through the Alien Property Act.[53] The fact that from then on Syntex's operations "depended on a licensing agreement with the US Attorney General" made them ripe for an antitrust action. This action took place in 1956 when several U.S.-based drug manufacturers "brought Syntex's monopolistic practices to the attention of the U.S. Senate Subcommittee on Patents, Trademarks and Copyrights." The companies' successful argument was that Syntex had suppressed competition in steroid research, inflating the price of plant steroids to raise other firms' barriers to entry. Syntex realized that its practices would render it liable to a costly, public antitrust suit, and thus ceased preventing other firms from having access to the Mexican raw materials and the processing patents.[54]

After Syntex settled the antitrust suit, companies including Searle, Smith Kline, Schering, and Wyeth Laboratories began to "take over pre-existing Mexican laboratories and set up their own subsidiaries within Mexico."[55] The increased need for raw material changed the Mexican government's policy to one of getting directly involved. Gathering and drying the *Barbasco* and yam roots was a cash crop for Mexican peasant farmers, who then sold them, originally to Syntex and later to the other companies. The disconnect between material costs and pharma profits existed even at this entry point. Marks notes that by the 1970s, the farmers were paid about 5 dollars for every 250 kilos of plant material (2 U.S. cents per kilo) in which 250 kilos were used to make 1 kilo of steroids. By then, pharma companies were realizing a profit of about 40 dollars from each gram of synthetic progestin made from the *Barbasco* root.[56]

A competitor firm to Syntex and then Diosynth was Productos Esteroides, "founded in 1955 by Irving W. Sollins, former sales manager for Syntex in the United States."[57] The pattern of interlaboratory and interfirm competition and networking affected other giants of hormonal research including Gregory Pincus, who was a friend of Irving Sollins. Productos Esteroides was marketed in the United States by a company called Root Chemicals, of which Pincus was a shareholder.[58] Pincus had a parallel career in Massachusetts to Russell Marker's in Mexico, and the two had met in the 1940s.

Credit for the development of the Pill must be given to three groups. The first includes the Mexican-based researchers, including Russell Marker, Carl Djerassi, and Luis Miramontes, and the second to their U.S. counterparts, Gregory Pincus and John Rock. Carl Djerassi and Gregory Pincus, who announced the creation of steroid hormone contraceptives in 1952, are typically called the fathers of the Pill. The third group to be credited includes the brave women who funded and pushed for research on the Pill, including Margaret Sanger and Katherine McCormick.

Like Djerassi and Russell Marker, Gregory Pincus was a brilliant individual who often chafed at institutional constraints. The description of Pincus offered by James Reed and others is one of a committed biologist from his early days, who studied under a prominent geneticist, William Castle at Harvard. Pincus's 1927 doctoral dissertation, relevant to his later research, was about hereditary factors influencing rats' coat coloring.[59] By 1936, Pincus was successful in artificially activating rabbit ova through exposure to salt solutions or temperature changes. He was also successful at transplanting developing ova into female rabbits, where they continued to develop as embryos. Unfortunately, Pincus's experiments were large, broad-ranging, and "too complex to be carefully controlled or easily reproduced."[60] He was denied tenure at Harvard University, partially based on anti-Semitic attacks.

An article entitled "No Father to Guide Them" appeared in *Collier's* in 1937, in which the author J. D. Ratcliff stated that "Pincus' experiments fit in with the work of that hugely famous Portuguese Jew Jacques Loeb." Ratcliff also wrote that the result of Pincus's experiments would "bring the mythical land of the Amazons to life . . . where man's value would be precisely zero."[61] Pincus then decided to pursue a one-year research contract at Cambridge University, thus unfortunately moving his family directly into the path of Nazi aggression.

The only saving grace at this point of Pincus's career was to be found in Worcester, Massachusetts, where Pincus's Harvard colleague Dr. Hudson Hoagland had moved to Clark University in the 1930s as head of its biology department. A colleague of Pincus's at Cambridge University, Baron Nathaniel Rothschild, "a fellow investigator of the mechanisms of reproduction," gave Hoagland 2500 dollars in salary for 2 years to hire Pincus. The money was necessary since Hoagland had only been able to hire Pincus for a courtesy visiting (nonfaculty, unpaid) appointment in zoology at Clark University. Additional funding was secured from a New

York businessman named Harry Ittelson, and the Rockefeller and Macy foundations.[62]

Reed notes that "by 1943 at Clark there were fifteen members in Hoagland's
research group" and only Hoagland was paid by and directly affiliated with the
university. All the others were supported by individual and foundation funds,
including a large converted barn belonging to Hoagland's rented house on the
Clark campus. Hoagland paid for the latter.[63] Hoagland began testing an anti-
convulsant for Searle on his arrival at Clark University, and then connected Dr.
Pincus to the company, which was interested in hiring Pincus for his knowledge
of steroidal formulations. While Searle was mainly interested in having Pincus
do research on corticosteroids, Pincus seemed to be mainly interested in contraceptive research. To continue their research with no political interference,
Hoagland and Pincus founded the Worcester Foundation in 1944. The foundation was made possible in part by money from Searle, including more than one-
quarter of its 1946 research budget of 160,000 dollars.[64]

By 1949, U.S.-based pharma companies were starting to realize the benefits of
supporting steroidal hormone research, but still not because of interest in contraception. The chief reason was that in 1948, corticosteroids became widely
available when the Merck company isolated cortisone from acid bile. That same
year, cortisone was successfully used on rheumatoid arthritis sufferers at the Mayo
Clinic.[65] Virtually overnight, the basis for pharma companies' objections to funding steroidal hormone research for either being too risky or too unprofitable disappeared. On the other hand, the Comstock laws were still in effect. The Merck,
Upjohn, and Searle companies were key players in the domestic race to be the
first in producing cortisone cheaply and in mass quantities.[66] While pharma companies were increasingly willing to invest in and profit from the cortisone side of
steroidal hormone research, they were still quite strict on their allocations for
contraceptive research. For example, the Worcester Foundation received a total
of 110,000 dollars per year from the pharma companies during the 1951–1961
decade, "distributed among numerous research projects at the foundation."[67]
Also, "despite the increasing support of scientific research by the National Science Foundation and the National Institutes of Health, neither agency funded
any investigations in the reproductive sciences in the 1950s."[68]

Pincus had been hired by Searle to create cortisone from cholesterol. His pre-
ferred method was to pump synthesized steroids through the adrenal glands of
cows. While these experiments were successful, they were extremely expensive
due to the need for high amounts of cow adrenal glands.[69] By 1951, an Upjohn
biochemist was successful in using "microbes . . . in imitation of the fermenta-
tion processes used to manufacture penicillin and streptomycin."[70] Searle was
left stung by having been beaten by Upjohn, particularly when it was funding a

highly talented team of steroidal chemists. When in 1951 Pincus asked Searle's director of research, Albert Raymond, for funding to start a research program on the development of a contraceptive injection or pill, Raymond replied in a stinging letter, "you haven't given us a thing to justify the half-million we have invested in you. . . . You will get more only if a lucky chance gives us something originating from your group which will give us a large profit."[71]

By 1951, Dr. Pincus had identified his chief interest as contraceptive research. In 1950, Dr. Pincus received a small grant (3100 dollars) from Planned Parenthood to research the contraceptive potential of various steroidal hormones.[72] Pincus began researching oral contraceptives at Margaret Sanger's request and had been asking Searle for more potential contraceptive substances to research.[73] Pincus also worked with a chemist from Searle's steroid research program, Frank Colton, who had been at the Mayo Clinic for the groundbreaking cortisone trials. Colton had derived a new, more efficient process for synthesizing cortisone. While at Searle and working to "improve the biological profile of cortisone or hydrocortisone," Colton synthesized a progestogen that was equally active to the norethisterone created by Syntex's Djerassi.

OTHER KEY ACTORS IN PINCUS'S RESEARCH

While the Searle company was still hemming and hawing into the early 1950s, Pincus increased his scientific team at the Worcester Foundation. Two important scientists whom he recruited were Min-Chueh Chang and John Rock.[74] Chang interested Pincus because he was a brilliant chemist and interested in research on sperm. Pincus called Chang the "sperm man" and himself the "egg man."[75] Each was wedded to his own part of the contraception picture and downplayed the importance of the other scientist's view.[76] Dr. Chang began the first animal (rabbit) experiments to specifically develop an oral contraceptive on April 25, 1951, whereas previous research had officially not been about this but rather on regulating the menstrual cycle and preventing miscarriages.[77] While success was claimed by Pincus and Chang in 1952 after administering high doses of progesterone to rabbits and rats, the downsides were that injections were far more effective than the vaginal suppositories or oral pills that had also been tested. Pincus and Chang both doubted that women would be interested in receiving daily injections.

Dr. Pincus made connections with people who could help to test and fund an oral contraceptive. In addition to Margaret Sanger, the second person with whom Pincus connected was Dr. John Rock of Harvard University. Rock could be of significant help to Pincus and the Worcester Foundation in three ways. Rock was a clinical physician, unlike Pincus, and thus was authorized to conduct trials on human subjects. Second, Rock was a highly respected ob-gyn, a full professor

at Harvard, and on the staff of the Free Hospital for Women in Boston. Therefore, he was able to lend solid credentials to the relatively unknown Worcester Foundation.[78] Finally, Rock was a Roman Catholic who had broadened his
mind about the types of contraceptives he believed acceptable within marriage.
In 1931, Rock put his reputation on the line by signing a petition with 15 other
prominent Boston physicians urging the repeal of the Massachusetts law pro-
hibiting the sale of contraceptives. Risking excommunication, he was the only
Catholic doctor to take that public stance.[79]

In addition, Dr. Rock served on the AMA's committee on contraception in
the 1930s and wrote a 1931 article in which he criticized the lack of training of
Massachusetts ob-gyns in contraception.[80] Rock was viewed as a powerful ally
by Pincus, and thus Pincus selected Dr. Rock as the main face of the Worcester
Foundation's human trials because he was not Jewish. Pincus feared that the
selection of other Jewish doctors to represent the Worcester Foundation would
invite the same anti-Semitism he had experienced.[81]

After World War II, Rock adapted to the thinking of demographers and other
social scientists that better birth-control methods were needed in the world since
they viewed the world's expanding population as a threat. The proponents of
birth control at home in the United States and throughout the world often relied
on an argument based in liberal discourse about quality of life and family size.
While many have criticized people like Rock and Sanger for these arguments, the
larger advocacy context of trying to get birth control legalized and normalized in
the United States is often overlooked. There is a strong strand of criticism that
Margaret Sanger was a eugenicist, but most of those statements can be traced
back to the Catholic Church and conservative religious publishers and authors.
As noted by many, Sanger's catalyst for activism was the fact that her mother
died at an early age, weakened by 18 pregnancies. While Sanger attended meetings of birth-control advocates in Europe and India, often convened by societies
with eugenics in their name, she was doing this primarily to cement networks of
wealthy individuals who could be helpful to her group in the United States. As
noted by the Feminists for Choice website, Sanger never took the stance that
particular racial or ethnic groups did not deserve to reproduce, as erroneously
has been claimed.[82] To today's feminists, her most objectionable statements in
her early years were those advocating sterilization for the mentally ill. However,
her public stance against marriage incited the Catholic Church against her, and
many articles and books incorrectly tie her free love philosophy to a eugenicist
stance. Angela Franks's work is an example of the latter.[83]

In the 1940s, Rock and Pincus worked on separate projects but met up again
at a 1952 conference. Dr. Rock had been conducting tests on previously infertile
women in studies using a combination of progesterone and estrogen.[84] When the

treatment ended, the women became pregnant. Pincus urged Rock to run studies on a steroid hormone–based pill to inhibit ovulation. Since estrogen-containing pills had caused cancer in laboratory animals, their plan was to use pills containing only progestins. These were the formulations owned by Searle (norethynodrel) and Syntex (norethisterone or norethindrone), respectively. Pincus also set up a research design whereby women would only get the pills for 20 days per month to allow for a menstrual period to take place. During 1954 and 1955, Drs. Pincus and Rock ran studies at the Free Hospital for Women, in two different clinics there: the Fertility and Endocrine Clinic and the Reproductive Study Center.[85] The studies were considered a success, in that the steroids inhibited ovulation and enabled 14 percent of the volunteers to become pregnant after they stopped taking the drugs.[86]

In 1955, two more sets of studies were attempted. The successful one was unfortunately conducted on involuntary subjects, 12 female and 16 male patients at the Worcester State Hospital who had been diagnosed as psychotic. A public study calling for volunteers would have violated the Comstock law still in effect in Massachusetts. For the first time, Pincus and Rock tested the effects of norethynodrel and an estrogen–progestin combination on the women's reproductive systems in general. Despite the small number of participants, this study became the baseline for the "long-term administration of 19-nor steroids in humans."[87] That same year, an attempted study on 23 female medical students at the University of Puerto Rico failed due to the onerous requirements of regular testing of body temperature, chemicals released in urine, and endometrial tissue (a particularly painful procedure) so as to prove ovulation timing.

By 1956, Pincus and Rock concluded that they were ready for phase 3 testing, after having concluded successful tests on laboratory animals and volunteers under controlled conditions. The third phase required testing of large numbers of voluntary subjects outside the controlled clinical environment. A workable framework was found in Puerto Rico, where both Rock and Pincus had contacts at the university's medical school. One hundred women from a housing project of the Rio Piedras suburb of San Juan were willing to participate under the direction of Dr. Edris Rice-Wray, a female physician from the university medical school who was also affiliated with the Public Health Department and Family Planning Association.[88] In Puerto Rico, as in Mexico, despite the prevalence of the Catholic religion, officials were willing to look the other way if persuaded that course of action would provide greater benefit. Women and officials were interested in controlling fertility on the highly populated island. The compound tested there was Searle's norethynodrel (10 mg) to which a small percentage of synthesized estrogen, mestranol (1.5%) had been added. The market name of this pill was Enovid. A high dosage of progestin was necessary to prevent ovulation, and the addition of mestranol prevented breakthrough bleeding. In his final reports, Pincus did not mention estrogen's cancer link previously found in laboratory animals.[89]

Enovid proved to be nearly completely effective as a contraceptive, by inhibiting ovulation as it was supposed to do. A few pregnancies were reported during the experiment, but were explained away as women's failure to consistently take Enovid. About 17 percent of the women experienced side effects such as nausea, headaches, and dizziness, leading Dr. Rice-Wray to conclude that Enovid probably needed to be refined for long-term use.[90] The secretary of health in Puerto Rico as well as some journalists opposed the neo-Malthusian nature of the Pill. Life was made so uncomfortable for Dr. Rice-Wray that in 1956, she left Puerto Rico to work for the World Health Organization in Mexico.[91]

When the FDA did approve Enovid in 1957 for menstrual disorders and as a contraceptive in 1960, it only did so on the basis of short-term use, for a time frame of less than one year.[92] In a form of a half-hearted denial as to what Searle researchers had been doing, the company told its shareholders' meeting in 1957 (subsequently reported in *Time*) that "some of the most hush-hush research has been pursued in dozens of laboratories in the effort to find a contraceptive pill." The article also mentioned Searle was soon to release a drug for menstrual problems that also inhibited ovulation.[93] While Searle claimed ownership of the pill at that point, it had consistently refused to be associated with its researchers either by acknowledging them or providing the required levels of funding. Searle bought two dedicated sources of plant steroids, the Productos Esteroides company and its U.S. marketing company Root Chemicals, in 1957.[94]

As of 1960, there had not been any long-term trials for Enovid. When she left Puerto Rico in December 1956, Dr. Rice-Wray sent Dr. Pincus what was then the most complete set of data then available, on 221 women comprising a total of 47 years of pill taking.[95] However, this was the dataset that Searle presented to the FDA as meeting the safety criterion in 1957 (for menstrual disorders) and 1960 (for contraception). The efficacy criterion was not added until the Kefauver Amendments of 1962.[96]

THE REAL FUNDING PICTURE

There are two women whose long-term efforts were indispensable to the Pill's development. They were Margaret Sanger and Katherine McCormick. Sanger was strongly formed by her experiences as a child, where she grew up as a daughter, one of six children of Irish immigrants. Her father, Michael Higgins, was described as rigid. Anne Higgins, Margaret's mother, ultimately bore 18 children (11 of whom lived) and died of tuberculosis and cervical cancer in her 40s. Michael Higgins was a stonecutter in the upstate factory town of Corning, New York, strongly committed to socialist and anarchist causes, transmitting those values on to Margaret. While Margaret believed in those values, she also appears to have innately been a feminist. Her feminist stances were imbued with her upbringing, since her mother consistently delivered 10-pound plus babies (and Margaret helped deliver a 14-pound sibling at the age of 8). While her mother died young, "her father lived to the age of eighty-four . . . and Margaret never got over the contrast."[97]

In the late 1890s, Sanger decided to go to nursing school at White Plains Hospital, a newly licensed facility. It has been described as a drafty building with no plumbing or central heating. Sanger took to nursing easily, becoming head nurse in the women's ward and married William Sanger, whom she had met in New York. While she found the architect an agreeable, progressive companion, she had no desire to rush into marriage. However, Mr. Sanger had other ideas and procured a minister and four witnesses without her knowledge, and the marriage took place in 1903.[98] Margaret Sanger was pregnant within six months, and gave birth to a son. She had also contracted tuberculosis from her mother, she believed, an ailment that plagued her for 23 years, by appearing in the glands of the neck, breast, and armpits and spots on the lungs, until her infected tonsils were taken out in 1920.

In 1910, Margaret and William attended a Socialist lecture in Yonkers, New York, which by all accounts provided an awakening for Margaret.[99] Margaret Sanger's activist life can be divided into two halves. The first was in New York City between the late 19th century through World War I, in which she functioned as a fairly radical activist and befriended Communists and anarchists such as Emma Goldman, Jack Reed, William Haywood, and Alexander Berkman.[100] During this first part of her activist life, she advocated free love and contraception for everyone, consistent with her friends' views.

Margaret participated in Socialist and Communist actions, including the famous Bread and Roses strike in Lawrence, Massachusetts, in 1912 and one in Paterson, New Jersey, in 1913. She also understood the "purely masculine reasoning of most radicals." Instead, she believed that the lack of women's control over reproductive decisions was "not at least partially responsible, along with industrial injustice, for the widespread misery of the world."[101] Sanger, a canny social movement entrepreneur and political activist, understood that to be effective, it was "necessary to concentrate on the one object to the exclusion of everything else."[102] In short, Sanger's life was one of creating a U.S.-based and then globally based social movement that would put women's needs for contraception and reproductive autonomy first.

Just as most of the right-wing themes of the late 20th and 21st centuries are dusted off from late 19th-century anxieties over the place of women in the social hierarchy, the same is true of the left. Socialism was as uncomfortable with feminism in 1912 as in the 21st century, and it is easy to remember the fights of feminists to be heard in the Students for a Democratic Society in the 1960s and in the Civil Rights and then Black Power movements. Sanger also had to confront the intransigence of the middle of the political spectrum who disdained her single-issue approach. However, guided by politically savvy mentors, Sanger later learned to play the middle-class divisions, such as those related to immigration anxiety, to her advantage. But through World War I, Sanger was much more a bohemian and Socialist than a liberal, although after World War I she would champion the liberal strategy of change to the Comstock laws.

In pre–World War I years, Sanger was a maternity nurse on the Lower East Side and saw hundreds of cases of botched abortions, maternal deaths, and women begging for contraception. She also started her newsletter known as the *Woman Rebel*, in which the term "birth control" was said to appear for the first time.[103] The magazine also contained invective against the "Baptist Church, and those Christian Associations funded by the Rockefellers and others . . . to kill the spirit of the workers of America."[104] While the newsletter did not offer information about birth control and was thus Comstock-legal, most issues were banned by the New York Post Office. In August 1914, Mrs. Sanger was indicted on nine counts of violating the Comstock Act by purportedly sending birth-control information through the mails. This made her liable to a 45-year sentence. After trying for a postponement of her trial that was futile, Sanger left the United States in 1914 leaving her husband to take care of their children. Right after she left, Comstock perpetrated a stealth attack on the household, calling on William Sanger and asking him to buy a copy of the birth-control pamphlet Margaret had had printed (and released while on her way to England aboard ship), called *Family Limitation*. William Sanger was later jailed one month for this action.[105] While in the United Kingdom, she practiced free love and concluded she really did not love William Sanger, and learned as much about mechanical methods of birth control (such as the diaphragm, then being tested in Europe) as she could.

When she returned, she was ready to continue her work for contraception, and was able to do so since the 1914 indictment was made to go away. Sanger and her sister Ethel Byrne opened the first birth-control clinic in the United States in 1916 with 50 dollars. The clinic was located in Brooklyn, New York and in the first 10 days of the clinic's operation, about 500 women arrived to get information on birth control. As Reed states, "for a fee of ten cents, Sanger and her sister showed applicants how to use diaphragms and cervical caps, condoms and other contraceptives."[106] Since this was an even more egregiously open flouting of the law than Sanger's birth-control pamphlets, there was a police raid on the clinic. Sanger was arrested in the raid, and sentenced to 30 days in the workhouse. Her appeal to the New York Court of Appeals was heard in 1918, which brought about the first potential crack in the Comstock laws by providing the justification for doctors to advise clients on contraception for the prevention or cure of disease, known as the *Crane* decision. Doctors were then allowed to give information about and prescribe contraceptives. Since Sanger was a nurse, she could not legally perform these practices and thus her conviction was upheld.

Sanger began to reach out to wealthy donors and to try to make her cause known among checkbook activists, in the manner of every effective social movement entrepreneur. She founded the monthly journal *Birth Control Review* in 1917 and the American Birth Control League (ABCL) in 1921. Her history with this organization and how it changed and ultimately became the Planned Parenthood Federation is that:

> Sanger served as president from 1921 until her resignation on June 12, 1928 over administrative differences with Acting President Eleanor Dwight Jones, a desire to concentrate on birth control research and clinical service at the Clinical Research Bureau, and her increased interest in international work. After her resignation, Sanger assumed full control of the CRB, renaming it the Birth Control Clinical Research Bureau (BCCRB), and severed all legal ties with the ABCL. In 1939, the ABCL merged with the BCCRB to form the Birth Control Federation of America, which in 1942 changed its name to the Planned Parenthood Federation of America.[107]

In 1921, the Sangers divorced and in 1922 Margaret married Noah J. Slee, the wealthy founder of the Three in One Oil Company. She insisted on separate apartments in the house they shared. Sanger backtracked from her previous denunciations of wealth and privilege. This probably had a great deal to do with her desire to fund her organizations and make contraceptive choice a universal reality in the United States, but it was a rather large shift in the space of about 10 years. While Sanger had denounced the Rockefellers in the *Woman Rebel,* Planned Parenthood would ultimately benefit hugely from their financial support. Slee himself could help Sanger in her endeavors since as a businessman, he owned a warehouse in Montreal and had the German manufacturers of the cervical caps and diaphragms ship these goods to his warehouse. He was assured of the necessity of this by a customs agent. Thus, the contraceptives would be packaged in Three-in-One cartons and driven into the United States. Slee also believed that contraceptive jellies then available were too expensive and unreliable, so he produced a lactic-acid-based jelly at his manufacturing plant in New Jersey.[108]

Sanger clearly wanted to establish a birth-control clinic in the United States that would pass legal muster, but a physician would have to be found to do so. In 1915, Sanger had met Marie Stopes, then a paleobotanist and marriage philosopher, at a birth-control conference held in London. Reed states that "Stopes had no knowledge of contraception until she was introduced to Sanger."[109] This is an interesting example of knowledge or policy transfer across the globe, since Marie Stopes International is one of the largest providers of contraceptives, abortion, and comprehensive sexuality information around the globe, with a particular presence in African nations. Planned Parenthood is the other major global provider of this nature. Reed suggests that Stopes's marriage to a wealthy aircraft manufacturer, and the fact she opened the first legal birth-control clinic in England in 1921, gave Sanger the push toward reframing her message in a more broadly based appeal (and perhaps her marriage to Slee in 1922).[110]

In 1923, Sanger had created the Clinical Research Bureau (CRB) as an arm's-length organization from the ABCL. This was required as the league was a membership organization and could not run a clinic. Sanger was also able to hire a doctor, Dorothy Bocker, who was from New York but was practicing in Georgia and desperate to return to New York. While she knew nothing of contraception, Sanger educated her on the Q.T. In its first year, the clinic (which was across the hall from the ABCL in its New York brownstone building) saw more than 1000 clients, most of whom were referred from across the hall.[111] From that time on, due to her international travels and notoriety, Sanger "had more invitations to lecture than she could accept at one hundred dollars a throw."[112] While Dr. Bocker was trying to work in a conscientious manner, she was criticized for the fact that in the CRB's first year she had used 13 different contraceptive regimens with 100 or fewer women in each group, with no systematic follow-up of clients. Women who did not return to the clinic for future appointments were strangely classified as a success, and Dr. Bocker did not compare failures against months of exposure to pregnancy.[113] However, Bocker's one major success was in unofficially establishing the high effectiveness of the spring-type diaphragm combined with spermicidal jelly.

Sanger decided not to renew Bocker's contract, and in revenge, the doctor took what records existed with her. Dr. Hannah Stone of New York volunteered to be the new doctor for the CRB, and performed a three-year follow-up study on the diaphragm and jelly series on more than 1100 cases. Dr. Stone kept meticulous records, and the clients were provided with follow-ups by a social worker. She published her findings in 1928, the first documentation that safe and effective mechanical contraception methods existed. Nevertheless, "organized medicine refused to take notice." Stone was forced to give up her association with the Lying-In Hospital due to her work for the CRB, and "for years membership in the New York County Medical Society was capriciously denied her."[114]

By 1930, Sanger was well-acquainted with the types of problems faced by Dr. Gregory Pincus in Worcester. Each was committed to a certain project, but also needed to constantly fund-raise to keep their endeavor going. In 1925, Sanger successfully asked the Rockefeller-funded New York Bureau of Social Hygiene for funds, got money from her millionaire husband, and from other philanthropists who were unwilling during Sanger's pre–World War I days. At the CRB clinic in 1930, 300 physicians were trained in contraceptive techniques. These physicians, who refused public association with the clinic, saw about 20,000 clients there.

At that point, the bureau was 17,000 dollars in debt. Sanger successfully raised 5000 dollars in funds from the Rockefeller Foundation even though continuing support of institutions was against the official foundation policy. Sanger helped start other clinics as well. In 1924, she had held a birth-control conference in Chicago to help Dr. Rachelle Yarros of Hull House to launch the second clinic in the United States. In 1930, she raised 5000 dollars to start a new birth-control clinic in Harlem, which was made a reality when the Julius Rosenwald Fund provided a matching grant. While community residents were ecstatic, physicians were not, somehow unrealistically viewing the clinic as competition for an as yet unmet need.[115] Sanger's clinics were repeatedly denied dispensary licenses, so she was operating in the interstices of the law. Her clinics were run by licensed women general practitioners.

From the *One Package* decision through the early 1940s, Sanger stepped back from running the birth-control movement. By 1940, "hundreds of thousands of women had participated in the movement by seeking contraceptive advice."[116] It is clear that by that time Sanger had spearheaded and galvanized the first wave of a reproductive-rights social movement in the United States and around the world.

Despite the fact that many doctors who were trained in contraception refused to publicly admit it, many physician-headed groups contested with Sanger for leadership of the U.S. pro-contraception movement. Two prominent examples included Dr. Robert Dickinson, who was an ob-gyn in Brooklyn who began his career there in the 1880s, and Dr. Clarence Gamble, heir to the Procter & Gamble fortune who graduated from Harvard Medical School in 1920 but proved much more adept as a researcher. Interestingly, both Dickinson and Gamble came from well-heeled backgrounds and in effect were the antithesis of Anthony Comstock, since both had families involved with the Young Men's and Women's Christian Associations (also favorite charities of the Rockefellers) yet were pro-contraception. Drs. Dickinson and Gamble and Margaret Sanger could be described spatially as a mobile of the planetary system, since at different points during the decades Sanger and Dickinson formed the center of the universe around which the other two lesser planets revolved. The axis would tilt depending on whether Sanger or Gamble wanted something from Dickinson, or Dickinson wanted something from Gamble.

Sanger and Gamble were distinguished not only by the class circumstances of their births, but also their view of what types of contraceptives women should and could have. Sanger made frequent research trips to Europe (and later Asia) and learned about cervical caps and diaphragms, and her clinics tested those in combination with spermicidal jelly. In contrast, based on no evidence, Gamble believed that women either could not or would not use barrier methods, and the studies he funded used only lactic-acid-based jelly or contraceptive foam (put on a wet sponge).[117] Dr. Dickinson was similar to Dr. John Rock in that both (like most physicians at the time) believed that contraception advice should only be given to married couples. Both had access to contributions from society ladies (and of course Gamble was self-funded throughout his life).

In 1916, Margaret Sanger had unsuccessfully asked Dickinson for his public support. He was opposed to that "promiscuous and self-promoting woman who was supportive of providing contraceptives to any woman who requested them." Like many of his cohort in the medical profession, he did not appreciate the decision-making structure at the CRB, in which Sanger and women physicians made policy.[118] Similarly, while Sanger did not care if recipients of contraceptives were married, the physicians usually did. Dickinson and Gamble never had a competitive relationship between them, unlike that with Sanger. The relationship between the two men was much more one of eminence grise–apprentice. After his Harvard Medical School graduation, Gamble was appointed as an assistant professor of pharmacology at the University of Pennsylvania. Knowing of Gamble's family wealth and his ability to support himself, Dickinson had hoped to hire Gamble as a contraceptive researcher, since most young men in the medical profession viewed that area as career suicide.[119] By the late 1920s, Gamble had washed out of his career at the University of Pennsylvania, due to an inconsistent work ethic. However, since he was to the manor born, Gamble was good at cultivating and retaining connections, particularly those of influential people. One colleague who was to ultimately prove central to the birth-control movement was Stuart Mudd, who had been a friend of Gamble's while they were undergraduates at Princeton and then fraternity brothers at Harvard. By the mid-1920s, Mudd was a microbiologist at the University of Pennsylvania and the head of the Birth Control Federation in Pennsylvania, a state notoriously resistant to progressive views on contraception.[120]

Reed notes that having heard that Sanger was about to open a second birth-control clinic in 1922 (with an obscure woman doctor in charge), Dickinson accelerated his efforts and got some wealthy women to fund an organization that would be headed by him, the Committee on Maternal Health. This organization was founded in 1923, the same year as the CRB. Dickinson enlisted the aid of other physicians, which was easy for him as a credentialed male, to conduct research on contraception, sterility, and abortion.[121]

After the end to his University of Pennsylvania career, Clarence Gamble moved to Milton, Massachusetts with his wife in 1937. He was able for much of his career to claim affiliation with either the committee (Dickinson's group), the ABCL (Sanger's association), or both. Gamble went to great pains to stay in good graces with Dickinson, since he likely felt that Dickinson had a greater potential for acceptance as a leader of the contraceptive cause than Sanger. First, he asked Dickinson and the Committee on Maternal Health to commit to a joint project to open a birth-control clinic in Gamble's hometown of Cincinnati, in honor of his mother who had just recently passed away. The committee was happy to oblige. Gamble's second action to keep himself in Dr. Dickinson's favor was to establish and fund the Robert Dickinson Research Fellowship in Chemistry at New York University in 1935. Gamble arranged for the distribution of the studies by its pro-contraception tenants.[122]

In addition to the Committee on Maternal Health and the ABCL, Gamble was given official status by the group created by microbiologist Stuart Mudd and his wife Emily, who had met Margaret Sanger and Dr. Hannah Stone when she worked at the Rockefeller Institute. When they moved to Pennsylvania in the 1920s, they were "appalled to find no birth control clinics available" and so created the Committee for Maternal Health Betterment, which opened the first clinic in the state in 1929.[123] The Mudds hired Gamble to test the efficacy of various contraceptive jellies. Within 5 years, 8 more clinics had been opened in the state, costing 10,000 dollars with about a third of that coming from patient fees. Gamble and other donors contributed the rest.

In addition, Gamble had the means and interest to fund contraceptive studies, but with the unusual and intrusive requirement for his involvement. He was quite entrepreneurial in tapping into existing frameworks and attempting (either successfully or not) to co-opt control of them. One federal government action ultimately proved helpful to Gamble. The legislation was Title V of the 1935 Social Security Act, which allocated an unprecedented 5.5 million dollars (in 1936 dollars) to state maternal and child health programs.[124] Hazel Moore, a suffragist movement veteran and former Red Cross relief administrator and lobbyist for Margaret Sanger's National Committee on Federal Legislation for Birth Control, seized on the opportunity. She suggested to Dr. Gamble that he lobby the Children's Bureau to allocate some of the funding to contra-ceptive research. Due to personality conflicts involving Margaret Sanger, this money was not released until the war effort, when more women were needed to work.

Two of Gamble's studies took place in rural Virginia and North Carolina, where public health services (i.e., distribution networks) already existed and he could control the methodology and report the results. Reed states that Gamble's first project in Logan County, occurring between 1936 and 1939, was "the most extensive and sophisticated field trial of a chemical contraceptive ever com-pleted in the US."[125] Gamble paid for a nurse to be flown in from Philadelphia and for the cost of the jelly distributed. Ortho Pharmaceutical donated the jelly at cost, an event in the 1930s that Pincus and others in the 1950s seeking fund-ing and steroids for research would likely envy. While Dickinson's Committee on Maternal Health had voted to stay out of routine delivery of contraceptive services, Gamble got funding through them to study the case records. Sophisti-cated is a curious term to use for a birth-control method that could not possibly succeed (jelly with no cervical barrier in place) and with no doctors on site.

Gamble frequently clashed with the leadership of the ABCL (including Sanger), and later the International Planned Parenthood Federation (IPPF) and the Population Council.[126] The league was very firm on having its methodology followed, as formulated and directed by the New York Office. Sanger had gone to jail, written books, and travelled around the world in order to perform studies on the efficacy of what she believed medically to be the best method, the female bar-rier methods augmented by spermicidal jelly. Very strangely, the league's medical director approved Gamble's study in West Virginia, believing that due to many unattended childbirths, the rural women would have severe uterine prolapses, making them unfit for studies using diaphragms and caps. Clearly, that sort of study would be impossible without the presence of a doctor.

Gamble's next study was commissioned in North Carolina, where the infra-structure again proved feasible. The assistant director of the State Board of Health, Dr. George Cooper, was quite amenable to a nonpublicized study where Gamble provided all the funding. Gamble was also able to send a nurse, Elsie Walkop, as he had done in the West Virginia study. In the one-year North Caro-lina study, foam powder was prescribed more than two-thirds of the time while the diaphragm and jelly method was prescribed less than one-third of the time. Still, the study was deemed a success, and North Carolina became the first state to include contraception in its public health program. Six other states in the south, targeted and funded by Gamble, soon followed suit. In 1942, following these successes and lobbying of the Child Health Bureau, the U.S. Public Health

Service ruled that Title V money could be used to provide family-planning programs by the states.[127]

Another success of Gamble's was found in Puerto Rico, 20 years before Drs. Pincus and Rock conducted their study there. In May 1935, the Puerto Rico Emergency Relief Administration had begun a program of contraceptive distribution, discontinued due to Catholic lobbying. Gamble sent Mrs. Phyllis Page, an employee, to Puerto Rico to interview Dr. Ernest Gruening, administrator of the Puerto Rican Reconstruction Administration (and future senator from Alaska). As with Dr. Cooper in North Carolina, Dr. Gruening admitted that a low-key, off-the-radar program privately funded by Dr. Gamble would likely achieve success. Characteristically, Gamble took unilateral action when approaching Sanger's league about sending Phyllis Page to Puerto Rico as an official ABCL representative, and to hire the distinguished obstetrician Dr. Jose Belaval who had been instrumental in the island's birth-control effort at a Gamble-funded salary of 200 dollars per month. The ABCL had a fairly explosive reaction to Gamble's initiative, and refused to agree with naming Page as an official representative. The bottom line was that Dr. Belaval was happy to have Mrs. Page's help and quite soon the two had formed an organization dedicated to women's and children's health, a copy of the organization Mrs. Page had started in Kentucky.[128] Over time, a network of 23 privately funded clinics was established in Puerto Rico. Legislation and test cases followed that, among other things, established the right in Puerto Rico (as established in the United States by the 1918 *Crane* decision) for physicians to prescribe contraceptives, and later established the compatibility of Puerto Rico's contraceptive regime with the Congressional changes of 1971.

After having turned down Margaret Sanger's request for help in 1916, Dr. Dickinson by 1924 sent his committee members into her clinic to make a surprise inspection. There, they availed themselves of the only consistent data source on the success of the diaphragm and jelly combination. Dickinson was impressed enough by the methods and data that by 1925 he had agreed to join a board of directors for the CRB (although the state board turned down the license application). While he conducted numerous attempts to have medical men take control of the bureau (all of which failed due to self-interest of the male physicians), Dr. Dickinson joined the first advisory board of the bureau in 1930.[129]

Disappointingly, after Sanger's strategy and effort to make the *One Package* decision happen in 1936, which interpreted Section 305 of the 1930 Smoot-Hawley Tariff Act as providing physicians legal cover under which to prescribe contraceptives, the men of the movement turned on her. The new line was that Margaret Sanger and her feminist colleagues in the New York City ABCL and CRB should step aside and let the real experts become the spokesmen of the birth-control movement. Since the AMA had approved of contraception in 1937, it is clear that doctors wanted to muscle in on a lucrative practice (250 million dollars per year in the 1930s).[130] Hazel Moore of the ABCL had proposed the strategy to Gamble of lobbying the federal government to include contraception as an approved expenditure for states under Title V. Gamble and other doctors from Dickinson's Committee on Maternal Health decided however that the birth-control movement needed to be taken away from Margaret Sanger because she was too radical and that moderation was needed in order to persuade the federal government to include family planning in public health funds. The claim put forth by the Gamble faction and reiterated by the mediator brought in to help discussions in the organization was that Sanger was too divisive and that competition for funding between the ABCL and the CRB were due to Sanger. He ignored the consistent lack of support and interest demonstrated by the male medical profession for nearly 30 years. Quite rightly, Sanger felt her movement had been hijacked by the medical men, but recognized that Gamble's money was needed to keep her organizations going.

The Gamble–Rose faction proposed a merger of the two organizations founded by Sanger into the seemingly less-offensive Birth Control Federation of America in 1939 with Rose appointed as its acting director, where he stayed until 1948. Rose proved to be a treacherous ally, for while he had pushed Sanger out for Gamble and his friends, he then turned around and pushed Gamble out in 1942. In 1942, Rose suggested a name change to Planned Parenthood Federation of America (PPFA) to dissociate from any perceived eugenicist taint and to sell the federal government on the need to fund family planning in the states. That particular policy was successful through the Public Health Service decision in 1942. Other successes from co-opting Sanger's organization were the nationalization of the movement so as to remove it from the control of Sanger's colleagues in New York City and to broaden the funding base. The funding base was widened, a more universal standard of practice for clinics across the United States was set, and "the group got a respectful hearing in high professional circles and from administrators in Washington."[131] Reed notes that the downsides included the fact that by 1950 the revenues were far less than what Rose had promised (a discretionary budget of 168,000 dollars for the year) and that the organization had seemingly become just another voluntary health organization with no real ability to influence policy.

Sanger's next direction came when a colleague in Sweden organized a birth-control conference in Stockholm, for leaders of the movement. From that conference came the determination to work for an internationally-based pro-contraceptive organization. An interim committee was struck, known as the International Planned Parenthood Committee, and Sanger got one of her long-term fund-raising and political action contacts, Dorothy Brush from the previous legislative campaign to underwrite an office for the committee. Brush was a Margaret Sanger supporter and worked in the office with her.[132] Moreover, Mrs. Brush became the secretary of the committee, and the Brush Foundation, which she controlled, contributed to the 1952 birth-control conference in Bombay at which the IPPF was launched. In order to avoid the demands from the PPFA for 15 percent of the contributions raised, the IPPF set up a tax-privileged arrangement with the Brush Foundation whereby IPPF contributors could give the money solely to that organization.[133] By the late 1950s, IPPF would become the leader in global reproductive health, including contraceptive and abortion counseling and provision, with Sanger's role unquestioned.

Through her international travels and then work with IPPF, Sanger came to believe that an anovulant pill was the next necessary step forward in contraception. On June 8, 1953, Sanger brought her friend Katherine McCormick to meet Dr. Pincus at the Worcester Foundation. McCormick was heir to the International Harvester fortune through marriage to Stanley McCormick, who died in 1947. McCormick decided at that point to fund Pincus and the Worcester Foundation's contraceptive research exclusively to a tune of 150,000–180,000 dollars annually until her death in 1967. This may be compared with the entire pharma industry's funding support of all the different projects at the Worcester Foundation at a level of 111,000 dollars annually from 1951 to 1961.[134] There is no doubt that McCormick's generous, stable funding enabled Pincus and Rock to expedite their research and the production of the pill. When it was clear that there was money to be made from this formulation (and from steroid hormones for cortisone), Searle was suddenly interested and back in the picture. In 1957, when Enovid was only being sold for menstrual disorders, Searle realized an annual profit of 37 million dollars from the pill. In 1964, due to market competition, that figure had dropped to 24 million dollars for the year, for which neither Dr. Pincus nor the Worcester Foundation received any royalties.[135]

FDA APPROVAL FOR NORETHISTERONE (SYNTEX) AND NORTHYNODREL (SEARLE) AND LATER ISSUES

Syntex's CEO Carl Djerassi and his coresearcher Miramontes filed the patent application on norethisterone in November 22, 1951 and Frank Colton of Searle filed his for northynodrel on August 31, 1953. The result was that "northynodrel was officially patented in November 1955, six months ahead of norethisterone (May 1956)."[136] While Marks believes that perhaps the U.S.-based Searle was more familiar with the levers of the U.S. bureaucracy and could navigate that framework more efficiently, she also shows that through the early 1970s, the "patents issued for the principal progestogens used in oral contraceptives" tended to be approved earlier when submitted by a U.S.-based company than one based abroad. On one hand, this is likely an indicator of the U.S. governmental process trying to foster U.S. entrepreneurialism, but on the other, it does smack of protectionism and parochialism. Syntex had a harder time getting its progestin-based norethisterone pill on the market for contraceptive purposes. In 1957, Syntex's progestin-only pill Norlutin was approved by the FDA for marketing for hormonal and menstrual disorders just as Enovid was. However, Syntex was a small company and faced other problems already solved by Searle. Originally, Syntex had tried to work with Parke-Davis, which had a very conservative marketing policy in the 1950s. Syntex did not have the means to sell norethisterone on its own and thus had to search for a lager pharma partner. Syntex later partnered with the Ortho division Johnson & Johnson to sell its pill, called Ortho-Novum (or Novin), which was made available for contraceptive purposes in 1963. Ortho-Novum was a combination of norethisterone–estrogen mestranol pill. As Marks notes, other pills approved in 1964 were Norlestrin and Norinyl, with a combination of norethisterone compounds with the synthetic estrogen compounds ethinylestradiol and mestranol.[137] In 1966, Gedeon Richter released (or re-released, depending on what one believes about its prior activities during the 1940s) Infecundin in Hungary.

In the 1960s, Searle conducted tests to win FDA approval for pills containing a lower dose of progestin. They tested pills at 2.5 and 5 milligrams, which were approved with no apparent hitches. By 1962, Searle had received reports of 132 women developing blood clots and 11 deaths but claimed that there was no link to the pill.[138]

Marks has shown that after Searle received FDA approval to sell the 10-milligram Enovid as a contraceptive in 1960, the domino effect of contraceptive drug formulation by other companies was quite rapid. For example, in 1964, Wyeth developed the compound norgestrel, "the first progestogen to be made from a total chemical synthesis."[139] After being licensed to Schering, norgestrel was used to make levonorgestrel, which is the chemical compound in Plan B, the morning-after pill. By 1973, between 25 and 30 different types of contraceptive pills had been developed, reports Marks, which included the fact that different brand names were used around the world for the same substance.[140] The number had jumped to 430 by 1992, reminding us of Philip Hilts's statements about the development of me-too drugs just so companies can make money.

By the early 1970s, largely due to feminist lobbying, the Searle formula of northynodrel, containing the intrinsic estrogen component that induced blood clots, was out of favor in the international market. Lobbying included the publication of activist Barbara Seaman's 1969 book, *The Doctors' Case against the Pill*, and feminist organizing and presence at the following Senate hearings conducted by Senator Gaylord Nelson of Wisconsin. Interestingly, the radical feminist DC Women's Liberation Group, formed around the issue of safe and legal abortion, came to the hearings and disrupted them by asking why the only witnesses called were male (and the Senate committee was all male). Seaman was not called on to testify; only male doctors were. Representatives of the pharma industry had been invited but none chose to attend.[141] The upshot of the two rounds of hearings was that inserts in the pill packages were agreed on by the FDA; however, the medical profession opposed them as interfering in the doctor–patient relationship. Ms. Seaman pointed out that most patients she interviewed who received the pill from physicians in private offices as opposed to public clinics were never informed of the risks posed by the Pill, especially Searle's northynodrel compound.[142]

In 1966, the Advisory Committee on Obstetrics and Gynecology of the FDA released its *Report on the Oral Contraceptives*. Dr. Roy Hertz, a committee member whose early work had influenced many others on steroid hormone research, issued an addendum to the report focusing on three principal health risks he believed to be innately tied to the Pill: cancer, blood clots, and reproductive defects from ova exposed to the Pill.[143] Despite his prominence and history in that particular field, the majority reported finding "no adequate scientific data at this time proving these compounds unsafe for human use." The FDA grudgingly agreed to put these into the Pill's package inserts in 1970, but only one disorder, blood clotting, was mentioned. The first draft had included risks from blood clots; the final draft did not. The pamphlet described 5 side effects (as opposed to the original proposed 25) for which women should seek doctors' care.[144] In 1977, the FDA released patient information requirements for women on estrogen (hormone-replacement) therapy, and in response, the Pill's patient insert was strengthened to be consistent with those of other products containing estrogen.[145]

Ultimately, with so many different types of pill choices developed after the 1960s, including sequential pills that limited progestin and estrogen exposure to 21 days of the menstrual cycle, women still stayed loyal to the Pill, particularly in the Global North. As of today, hormonal contraceptives (including Depo-Provera) and male or female sterilization are the most popular contraceptive methods.

CONCLUSION

Many of the themes, strategies, and legislative frameworks that were used by contraception opponents starting in the late 19th century have been used by social conservatives to curtail women's reproductive autonomy into the

21st century. Tarrow's political process model was also relevant to this discussion, but more regarding the absence of women's relationship to allies and the state than in a positive sense. While Margaret Sanger fought from 1914 to 1936 to undo Comstock prohibitions, the resulting *One Package* decision of 1936 gave fodder to the male physicians and their allies to move in and seize control of her organizations, with the help provided by Clarence Gamble and his money. Therefore, while women should have had greater access to the state under the post-1936 policy regime, they did not, since the court decision only spoke to the rights of physicians. Women and men in the pro-contraceptive movement had to continue fighting through the second half of the 20th century, including Estelle Griswold from Planned Parenthood in New Haven, before the 1965 *Griswold* and 1972 *Eisenstadt* decisions made birth-control access a privacy right for all.

Institutionalist theories were also helpful frames for this discussion, including those of discursive institutionalism and historical institutionalist processes of conversion and layering. Unfortunately, for the discussion of how the pill came to be formulated, most of these processes were controlled by conservatives. The only feminist aspect was the continued work of Margaret Sanger to make contraception in general available, and to work with Katherine McCormick and Gregory Pincus specifically on the pill. One example of layering was helpful to women when Title V of the 1935 Social Security Act was passed and interpreted in 1942 to make contraception funding available in the states.

NOTES

    1. Wolfgang Streeck and Kathleen Thelen, eds., *Beyond Continuity: Institutional Change in Advanced Political Economies* (London: Oxford University Press, 2005), 1–39 and Jacob S. Hacker, "Policy Drift: The Hidden Politics of US Welfare State Retrenchment," in Streeck and Thelen, *Beyond Continuity*, 40–83.

    2. Nicola Beisel, *Imperiled Innocents: Anthony Comstock and Family Reproduction in Victorian America* (Princeton, NJ: Princeton University Press, 1997), 39–41 and Leslie J. Reagan, *When Abortion Was a Crime: Women, Medicine and the Law in the US, 1867–1973* (Berkeley, CA: University of California Press, 1998).

    3. Daniel P. Carpenter, *The Forging of Bureaucratic Autonomy: Reputations, Networks, and Policy Innovation in Executive Agencies, 1862–1928* (Princeton, NJ: Princeton University Press, 2001), 84–88.

    4. Donald Critchlow, *Intended Consequences: Birth Control, Abortion and the Federal Government in Modern America* (Oxford: Oxford University Press, 2001), 50–112.

    5. James Reed, *The Birth Control Movement and American Society: From Private Vice to Public Virtue* (Princeton, NJ: Princeton University Press, 1984), 102.

6. Jennifer Lee, "James H. Scheuer, 13-Term Congressman, Is Dead at 85," *New York Times*, August 31, 2005, http://www.nytimes.com/2005/08/31/nyregion/31scheuer. html and Wendy McElroy, *Sexual Correctness: The Gender-Feminist Attack on Women* (Jefferson, NC: McFarland and Company, 2006), Chapter 3.

7. United States Representative to the United Nations George H. W. Bush, Jr., "Foreword," in *World Population Crisis: The United States Response,* ed. Phyllis Tilson Piotrow (New York: Praeger, 1973), viii.

8. Daniel J. Kevles, "The Secret History of Birth Control," *New York Times*, July 22, 2001, http://www.nytimes.com/2001/07/22/books/the-secret-history-of-birth-control. html?pagewanted=all&src=pm.

9. Lori Klatt Maurice, "Stamping Out Indecency the Postal Way," March 8, 2004, 1–14, http://academic.evergreen.edu/k/klalor09/post%20office%20censorship%20home. htm, unpublished paper.

10. Mary Ware Dennett, *Who's Obscene?* (New York: The Vanguard Press, 1930), 214, cited in Maurice, "Stamping Out Indecency."

11. Maurice, "Stamping Out Indecency" and Nicola Beisel, *Imperiled Innocents: Anthony Comstock and Family Reproduction in Victorian America* (Princeton, NJ: Princeton University Press, 1997), Chapters 1, 2, and 7.

12. Maurice, "Stamping Out Indecency," 4–6, 10–12; the case was *NY vs. Sanger,* 1918.

13. Reed, *The Birth Control Movement,* 120–21; the case was the Second Federal Circuit Appellate Court's decision, the *One Package* decision of 1936.

14. Wallace F. Jannsen, "The Story of the Laws behind the Labels," *FDA Consumer* 15, no. 5 (June 1981): 32, cited in Stephen J. Ceccoli, *Pill Politics: Drugs and the FDA* (Boulder, CO: Lynne Rienner Publishers, 2004), 58.

15. Raymond Ahearn, *US Trade Policy and Changing Domestic and Foreign Priorities: A Historical Overview,* CRS Report No. RS21657 (Washington, DC: Congressional Research Service, November 3, 2003), http://congressionalresearch.com/RS21657/ document.php?study=U.S.+Trade+Policy+and+Changing+Domestic+and+Foreign+Prio rities+A+Historical+Overview.

16. "1890–1933 Reform and Revenue," U.S. Government Printing Office, http:// www.gpo.gov/fdsys/search/pagedetails.action;jsessionid=Ky9gQQHFNvRVm15qsYPS M3n4Vpy2hmqLTmS8gKKQt7qJyzVMKGrC!-1164936703!2001895722?granuleId= GPO-CDOC-100hdoc244-15&packageId=GPO-CDOC-100hdoc244&fromBrowse=true, 215–71, 226–27.

17. "Medicare: AMA at New Orleans," *Time,* May 23,1932, http://www.time.com.

18. Senator Smoot's actions are described in Steve Charnovitz, "The Moral Exception in Trade Policy," 38 *Virginia Journal of International* Law 689 (Summer 1998), 266 and Eli Oboler, "Congress as Censor," *Library Trends* (July 1970): 64–73, http://www.ide als.illinois.edu/bitstream/handle/2142/6533/librarytrendsv19i1g_opt.pdf?sequence=1.

19. Reed, *The Birth Control Movement,* 121.

20. Ibid., 120.

21. Ibid., 239.

22. Daniel Carpenter, *Reputation and Power: Organizational Image and Pharmaceutical Regulation at the FDA* (Princeton, NJ: Princeton University Press, 2010), 3.

23. Theodore Lowi, *The End of Liberalism: The Second Republic of the United States* (New York: W. W. Norton and Company, 2009).

24. Center for Responsive Politics, www.opensecrets.org.

25. Marcia Angell, *The Truth About the Drug Companies: How They Deceive us and What to Do About It* (New York: Random House, 2005); Fran Hawthorne, *Inside the FDA: The Business and Politics behind the Drugs We Take and the Food We Eat* (Hoboken, NJ: J. Wiley, 2005); and Philip J. Hilts, *Protecting America's Health: The FDA, Business, and One Hundred Years of Regulation* (Chapel Hill, NC: University of North Carolina Press, 2003), 191–94.

26. Angell, *The Truth About the Drug Companies*, 216, ft. 27.

27. "Steroid Hormones," St. Edward's Computer Science, http://www.cs.stedwards.edu/chem/Chemistry/CHEM43/CHEM43/Steroids/Steroids.HTML.

28. Michelle Kerns, "What are Steroid Hormones?", eHow health, http://www.ehow.com/about_5047511_steroid-hormones.html.

29. Edward M. Graham and David M. Marchick, *US National Security and Foreign Direct Investment* (Washington, DC: Institute for International Economics, 2006), Chapter 1.

30. Lara V. Marks, *Sexual Chemistry: A History of the Contraceptive Pill* (New Haven, CT: Yale University Press, 2010), 41.

31. Ibid., 41–43.

32. Ibid., 43–45.

33. Ibid., 47.

34. Ibid., 47–48.

35. Ibid., 45.

36. Ibid., 58.

37. Ibid., 46–58.

38. Ibid., 64–65.

39. Ibid., 65.

40. Ibid., 65.

41. Ibid., 65.

42. Ibid., 34–35, 64–66.

43. Ibid., 61–67.

44. Ibid., 64.

45. Ibid., 67–69.

46. Ibid., 68–70.

47. Reed, *The Birth Control Movement*, 355.

48. Ibid., 355–56.

49. Marks, *Sexual Chemistry*, 71.

50. Ibid.

51. Reed, *The Birth Control Movement*, 327.

52. Marks, *Sexual Chemistry*, 83.

53. Reed, *The Birth Control Movement*, 357.

54. Ibid.

55. Marks, *Sexual Chemistry*, 84.

56. Ibid., 83–84.

57. Reed, *The Birth Control Movement*, 357.

58. Ibid.

59. Reed, *The Birth Control Movement*, 317–33; see also Marks, *Sexual Chemistry* and Elizabeth Siegel Watkins, *On the Pill: A Social History of Oral Contraceptives, 1950–1970* (Baltimore, MD: The Johns Hopkins University Press, 1998), Chapter 2.

60. Reed, 317–33.

61. J. D. Ratcliff, "No Father to Guide Them," *Collier's Magazine*, March 20, 1937, 19, cited in Reed, *The Birth Control Movement*, 323, ft. 21.

62. Reed, *The Birth Control Movement*, 325.

63. Ibid., 328–29.

64. Ibid., 329–31.

65. Ibid.

66. Ibid., 331.

67. Watkins, *On the Pill*, 25.

68. Ibid.

69. Reed, *The Birth Control Movement*, 327–29.

70. Ibid., 332.

71. Letter from Albert Raymond to Gregory Pincus, October 1951, cited in Reed, *Birth Control Movement*, 332–33, ft. 50.

72. Reed, *The Birth Control Movement*, 332.

73. Marks, *Sexual Chemistry*, 71.

74. Watkins, *On the Pill*, 27–29.

75. Marks, *Sexual Chemistry*, 90.

76. Ibid., 90–91.

77. Ibid.

78. Ibid., 93.

79. "The Pill: People and Events, Dr. John Rock (1890–1984)," Public Broadcasting Service (PBS), http://www.pbs.org/wgbh/amex/pill/peopleevents/p_rock.html.

80. Reed, *The Birth Control Movement*, 352.

81. Ibid.

82. "Let's Chat: Margaret Sanger and Eugenics," *Feminists for Choice*, October 14, 2009, http://feministsforchoice.com/lets-chat-margaret-sanger-and-eugenics.htm.

83. Angela Franks, *Margaret Sanger's Eugenic Legacy: The Control of Female Fertility* (Jefferson, NC: McFarland and Company, 2005).

84. Watkins, *On the Pill*, 29.

85. Ibid.

86. Ibid.

87. Watkins, *On the Pill*, 30.

88. Ibid., 31.

89. Ibid., 30–31.

90. Reed, *The Birth Control Movement*, 360.

91. Ibid.

92. Watkins, *On the Pill*, 32.

93. "Contraceptive Pill?", *Time*, May 6, 1957, 83, cited in Watkins, *On the Pill*, 42.

94. Reed, *The Birth Control Movement*, 357.

95. Ibid., 360.

96. Watkins, *On the Pill*, 32.

97. Ibid., 67–100.

98. Reed, *The Birth Control Movement*, 72–73.

99. Ibid.

100. Ibid., 75.

101. Ibid., 77–79.

102. Ibid., 96.

103. "On This Day, September 7, 1966: Margaret Sanger Is Dead at 82; Led Campaign for Birth Control," *New York Times*, September 7, 1966, Obituary, http://www.nytimes.com/learning/general/onthisday/bday/0914.html.

104. Reed, *The Birth Control Movement*, 86.

105. "On This Day."

106. Reed, *The Birth Control Movement*, 106.

107. "The Margaret Sanger Papers Project: Birth Control Organizations," http://www.nyu.edu/projects/sanger/secure/aboutms/bc_organizations.html.

108. Reed, *The Birth Control Movement*, 114.

109. Ibid., 112.

110. Ibid.

111. Ibid., 114.

112. Ibid., 113.

113. Ibid., 115.

114. Ibid., 115–16.

115. Ibid., 116–19.

116. Ibid., 123.

117. Drawn from Reed, *The Birth Control Movement*, Chapters 11 and 17.

118. Ibid., 175.

119. Ibid., 225.

120. Ibid., 229–31.

121. Ibid., 168.

122. Ibid., 235, 245.

123. Ibid., 233.

124. Ibid., 261–66.

125. Ibid., Chapter 19.

126. Ibid., 226.

127. Ibid., 254. The other southern states in which Gamble was successful included Alabama, Florida, Georgia, Mississippi, South Carolina, and Virginia.

128. Ibid., 259–60.

129. Ibid., 175.

130. Ibid., 239.

131. Ibid., 268.

132. Ibid., 290–91.

133. Ibid., 292.

134. Watkins, *On the Pill*, 25–26.

135. "Timeline: The Pill, 1951–1990," *Public Broadcasting Service (PBS)*, http://www.pbs.org/wgbh/amex/pill/timeline/timeline2.html.

136. Marks, *Sexual Chemistry*, 71–72.

137. Ibid., 76.

138. "Timeline: The Pill, 1951–1990."

139. Marks, *Sexual Chemistry*, 76.

140. Ibid., 76–77.

141. Watkins, *On the Pill*, 107–28.

142. Ibid., 127.

143. Ibid., 87.

144. Ibid., 122.

145. Ibid., 128.

4

U.S. Pro-Choice and Pro-Life Groups' Strategies since 1960

This chapter explains the pro-choice and pro-life movements' trajectories since 1960. There are two policy regimes covered, the first one a fairly short time frame from 1960 until 1973, when women's reproductive policy interests were aligned with the general government frame. The interest in both Democratic and moderate Republican administrations in global and U.S. population issues and aiding firms in those areas helped women to achieve national access to publicly-funded contraception. This was a significant development, even though women were only represented in single-digit percentages in Congress at the time. The symbol of the policy punctuation between the first period on reproductive drug policymaking in the United States and the second was the election of 1980, the start of a rolling realignment that continued through 1994 and the end of the George W. Bush administrations in 2008.[1] The Reagan Revolution brought in a new electoral coalition to the Republican Party, including many former Democrats among the ranks of blue-collar workers, Catholics, and Southerners. The domestic ethos of his administrations was to shrink the size of government, and although his project, like those of most conservative governments, was not successful at the national level, it was successful in other realms. The main examples of his success were a seemingly permanent devolution of social policy administration and funding to the states under the new federalism rubric, continued by President Bill Clinton.

PRO-CHOICE DOMINANCE AND ACTIONS
IN THE FIRST REGIME, 1960–1973

The boundaries of the period start with the FDA's approval of the Pill for contraceptive purposes in 1960 until the 1973 U.S. Supreme Court's *Roe v. Wade* decision. A third important event was the 1970 passage of Title X of the Public Health Service Act, which established a national system of publicly-funded clinics to provide reproductive health care. President Nixon was in full support of this measure, stating that "no American woman should be denied access to family planning assistance because of her economic condition. . . . This we have the capacity to do."[2] As Coleman and Jones have noted, the Title X–supported clinics provide services that are not reimbursable under Medicaid and commercial insurance plans. They also observed that Title X received 4 of its 6 largest appropriations increases during its first 10 years.[3] The second policy period has involved the continual erosion of women's rights to access contraception, comprehensive sexuality education, and abortion.

In the pro-choice coalition, the earliest well-known single-issue group was the National Association for Repeal of Abortion Laws (NARAL), formed by journalist Lawrence Lader, author Betty Friedan, and Dr. Bernard Nathanson in New York in 1968, around their successful attempts to repeal the abortion law of New York State. Lader's 1966 book, *Abortion,* was cited eight times in Justice Harry Blackmun's *Roe v. Wade* decision.[4] In 1973, after *Roe,* NARAL changed its name to the National Abortion Rights Action League and became the preeminent mass single-issue organization that fought mainly in legislatures, courts, and public opinion discourse to keep abortion safe and legal. In 1976, Lader left NARAL and formed his own organization, Abortion Rights Mobilization (ARM) to perform more niche-based actions without having to go through the bureaucratic structure that had developed at NARAL.

Lader had become interested in U.S. reproductive-rights policy by researching and writing a biography on Margaret Sanger, who while pro–birth control had been against abortion. That led Lader to become active in the fight to overturn abortion laws in his home state of New York and to write his 1966 book. The Planned Parenthood Federation of America (PPFA) was formed in 1942.[5] This website states that PPFA has "ninety-five locally governed affiliates across the US" and "more than 850 health care centers."[6] It also states that more than 90 percent of its clinic services are focused on preventive health care, including pregnancy prevention, and that 77 percent of its clients are at least 20 years old.

From a 21st-century point of view, information about the 1960s U.S. governmental consensus on contraception seems incredible:

> As a central element of the War on Poverty, President Lyndon Johnson singles out a lack of family planning as one of four critical health problems facing the nation: the U.S. Department of Health, Education, and Welfare creates a program to provide contraceptive services for low-income, married women. Amendments to the Social Security Act require that at least six percent of the annual appropriations for maternal and child health be earmarked for family planning and that family planning services be provided to public assistance recipients who request them. The U.S. Agency for International Development begins providing contraceptives as an integral part of its overseas development programs.[7]

During the Johnson and Nixon administrations, funds were provided to low-income women to access contraception. According to Critchlow, the bargain that was struck during the early 1960s was that the U.S. Catholic Church would not actively oppose public funding for birth control as long as those programs were voluntary and the Church could still preach against this chemical contraception in its parishes and advocate the rhythm method instead.[8] Critchlow further states that at that time, the U.S. Catholic hierarchy was mindful of the need to cultivate the American public during the Kennedy presidency and so was amenable to soft-pedaling its stance on contraception. One of the key people who helped broker this compromise was John D. Rockefeller III who founded and funded the Population Council, formed in 1952. The Population Council and the Rockefeller Foundation have been the source of funding for agricultural and chemical research around the world, and the provision of birth control globally and in the United States.

The Population Council was founded in 1952 by John D. Rockefeller III, brother of Nelson Aldrich Rockefeller who served as New York governor from 1959 to 1973, crucially during the time of the abortion liberalization legislation in 1968. Both shared an interest, like Margaret Sanger, in population control and population health. They also had extensive experience in Latin America: Nelson through appointments in the Truman and Eisenhower administrations in the State Department and National Security Council and John through his Population Council work in funding agriculture and pharma companies such as Procter & Gamble and Upjohn who tested their products there.

The Rockefeller fund supported Planned Parenthood and the Population Council through public appeals to women's autonomy. On the other hand, as some analyses note, Malthusian thought ran rampant through the Population

Council at certain points in its history. Both pro-choice and Malthusian views could end up in the same place, being pro-choice and allowing—largely off the public radar screen—the testing of contraceptives and agricultural products in Latin America and Puerto Rico by Upjohn and Procter & Gamble. Gamble is another family who made money in both chemical products and contraceptives. Its descendants founded the Pathfinder Foundation and have been involved with Planned Parenthood as well; for example, both Richard Gamble (Clarence's son) and his wife Nikki Nichols Gamble have worked with Planned Parenthood of Massachusetts. Critchlow also notes that soon in the 1960s, the Population Council felt too many strictures in providing birth control through the federal government's programs and quickly the PPFA became their major provider.

The International Planned Parenthood Federation (IPPF) was founded in Bombay, India in 1952 and at least two other internationally-based companies were formed in the 1960s and 1970s, funded through some combination of Rockefeller, Population Council, and Planned Parenthood money. These companies state on their websites that they exist to provide direct assistance to developing partnerships with private-sector pharma companies in the area of reproductive and sexual health. The earlier one founded in this manner is the Program for Appropriate Technology in Health (PATH).[9]

The PATH website adds that the company was originally formed as the Program for Introduction and Adaptation of Contraceptive Technology (PIACT), and its first full-scale international project, contracted with the United Nations Population Fund (UNFPA), was in China. The PATH website describes its work as "modernizing contraceptive factories and boosting production to keep up with the country's burgeoning population." At the same time, the organization was branching out into other Asian countries to promote the same type of activity. PIACT became known as PATH in 1980 and it is now active in more than 70 countries, receiving funds from the same types of foundations that support other reproductive-rights research and technologies. Other supporters include the Packard, Hewlett, Ford, MacArthur, Susan Buffett, Doris Duke, Soros, and Gates foundations.[10] The Soros and Buffett foundations have been helpful in replacing monies lost when Republican presidents revoke U.S. Agency for International Development and UNFPA funding. The Gates Foundation has been particularly important in working with the United Nations since the declaration of the U.N. Millennium Development Goals in 2000. Since Bill Gates's wife Melinda is Catholic, the fund does not support any abortion-related activities.[11]

Another reproductive health foundation is the Concept Foundation, which was involved in helping to secure funding and siting for developing RU-486

in China when no US-based company would license it and also helped
fund development of Plan B. The Concept Foundation was established in
1989 in Bangkok, Thailand, through funding from the UNFPA, UNDP,
WHO, Population Council, International Planned Parenthood Federation
and the World Bank to "create a mechanism through which WHO's rights
associated with an injectable contraceptive could be licensed to potential
producers in developing countries."[12]

This drug, Cyclofem, is largely based on the Depo-Provera formulary
owned by Pfizer with an addition of synthetic estrogen. The Concept Foundation's homepage states its multi-faceted pro-choice activities.[13]

Another group crucial to trying to maintain the pre-1980s expansive
reproductive-rights framework is the Guttmacher Institute, named for Dr. Alan
Guttmacher, the president of Planned Parenthood in the 1960s and 1970s. The
institute was founded in 1968 as the Center for Family Planning Program and
Development, to work with the Johnson and then Nixon administrations in
delivering publicly-funded contraception. The center was originally formed as a
"semi-autonomous division of PPFA."[14]

Another important pro-choice advocate at the national and particularly
international levels has been the Center for Reproductive Rights (CRR), which
changed its name in 2003 after being formed as the Center for Reproductive
Law and Policy in 1992. The original group was formed when feminist litigators
left the American Civil Liberties Union. The CRR works often in tandem with
the Guttmacher Institute, Planned Parenthood, and NARAL. It could best be
described as a legal defense fund for reproductive rights, on the national but again
especially on the international scale. On its website, the center states about its
mission that it "has used the law to advance reproductive freedom as a fundamental human right that all governments are legally obligated to protect, respect, and
fulfill."[15] The center has litigated and won important cases that, among other
things, forced the Bush administration to allow Plan B over-the-counter for those
18 years old and over in 2006, and Latin American governments to enforce their
own pro-choice laws.[16]

William Saletan uses a helpful schematic on both the pro-choice and pro-
life sides. He refers to purist groups as those who would not condone any sort
of compromise in their goals. On the pro-choice side, Saletan has characterized
NARAL (National Abortion Rights Action League) as being instrumentalist to
the exclusion of being purist on the choice issue, where he shows that in three
different electoral races, NARAL lined up twice behind the more conservative
candidate on abortion because they believed he could win. This happened in
their support of Doug Wilder in the 1989 Virginia gubernatorial election and

Al Gore versus the more liberal Bill Bradley in the 2000 presidential primaries. According to Saletan, for some odd reason, NARAL stayed out of the 1990 Georgia gubernatorial race where Andrew Young offered a much more liberal position than Zell Miller.[17]

Saletan has characterized the pro-life groups based on whether they are predominantly affiliated with the Catholic or Protestant Churches. In the former group, he includes the U.S. Catholic Conference, the National Right to Life Committee, the American Life League (ALL), and Feminists for Life. The more Protestant groups are the Christian Coalition, the Family Research Council (FRC; absorbed into Focus on the Family [FOF] in the late 1990s), Concerned Women for America (CWA), Eagle Forum, and the Traditional Values Coalition.[18] Saletan describes the purists in both pro-life and pro-choice sides as those who are not amenable to compromise, either in their rhetoric or in support of middle-ground legislation. In the pro-life coalition, Saletan describes the purists as those who could not sanction anything that would destroy life, typically the Catholic-affiliated groups, while the Protestant ones—more concerned with encouraging procreation inside the family and discouraging it outside those boundaries—might support a measure that the other group feared would promote abortion. Saletan distinguishes these Protestant groups as pro-family rather than pro-life purists.[19]

The fragile bargain that had enabled contraception to be provided without means to pay broke after *Roe v. Wade*.[20] As Lawrence Lader, founder of NARAL and ARM, wrote, the entire pro-choice community was surprised by the sweeping breadth of Supreme Court Justice Harry Blackmun's 1973 decision. Another crucial event happened in 1964, when U.N. Secretary-General U Thant accorded special status to the Vatican as a non-state Permanent Observer member of the governing Economic and Social Council. As Critchlow has noted, the *Roe* decision removed the willingness of the U.S. Catholic Church to remain a silent partner in the expansionist regime. Starting in 1980, under Ronald Reagan, the U.S. Catholics joined their fundamentalist Protestant counterparts in becoming Reagan Democrats.

DOMINANCE OF THE PRO-LIFE COALITION IN THE SECOND POLICY PERIOD AFTER *ROE V. WADE*

The institutional mechanisms of the second policy period have included the following. The first has involved the election of more social conservative legislators at all levels, and scaling back pro-choice federal appropriations for Title V of the Social Security Act and Title X of the Public Health Service Act regarding contraception. In the parlance of the historical institutionalists, this strategy has involved drift, whereby fewer women are covered under these systems than before.[21] It has been noted that "if appropriations had kept up with inflation since FY 1980, the program would be funded at $840.1 million rather than the FY 2010 funding level of $317.5 million . . . funding for Title X in constant dollars, taking inflation into account, is 62% lower today than it was 30 years ago."[22]

Key players among the pro-life groups that have worked on a single-issue basis to undo *Roe v. Wade* have included the National Right to Life Committee (The NRLC) and Americans United for Life (AUL).[23] The website of AUL states that it "was incorporated as the first national pro-life organization to counter, through national education, the growing threat of disrespect for human life." By 1975, it had added public-interest law as part of its work.[24] That of ALL says that it was "founded by Ms. Judie Brown in 1979 and is the largest grassroots Catholic pro-life education organization in the US."[25] The NRLC appears to favor working on legislation, while AUL is a litigating group, and the ALL describes itself as an educational organization.

There were two early victories for the NRLC and AUL. The first was that of the 1974 Church Amendment not to force providers to provide services against their consciences. The Guttmacher website notes that "almost every state has a policy explicitly allowing some health care professionals or certain institutions to refuse to provide or participate in abortion, contraceptive or sterilization services." Also, in states without explicit refusal clauses, anti-religious-discrimination laws may protect individual employees.[26] This strategy may certainly be considered a success for the pro-life movement in restricting the availability of services to women, as has been its intent.

Another such early policy win was that of the 1976 Hyde Amendment (later adopted by the bulk of the states) not to allow Medicaid funding for abortions except in the cases of rape, incest, or life endangerment. The Guttmacher Institute reports that 32 states follow the federal Hyde framework, and 1 state, South Dakota apparently in violation of federal law goes beyond it only to allow Medicaid funding in the case of the mother's life endangerment. Similarly, 17 states provide nearly full funding for Medicaid-eligible women, but 14 of them only after a court order was obtained.[27] The website of AUL states that it was a central actor in the litigation of the 1980 *Harris v. McRae* Supreme Court decision upholding the Hyde amendment.

Two other prominent members of the pro-life coalition since the 1970s include CWA and FOF. CWA states that it was galvanized to action in 1978, when founder Beverly LaHaye, wife of televangelist Tim LaHaye, was watching Betty Friedan, founder of the National Organization for Women on television. As CWA website states, "realizing that Friedan claimed to speak for the women of America, Beverly LaHaye was stirred to action. She knew the feminists' anti-God, anti-family rhetoric did not represent her beliefs, nor those of the vast majority of women."[28]

While CWA was initially engaged with anti–Equal Rights Amendment advocacy, along with Phyllis Schlafly's Eagle Forum, it joined the anti-contraception and anti-abortion fight in the 1980s. CWA appears to be as multi-issue and amorphous as Schlafly's Eagle Forum in that it will move from one issue to the next, where both are described as pro-family, anti-abortion, and anti-communist. In 1980, the LaHayes were named Co-Chairs of an alternative conference to the liberal White House Conference on Families. While CWA was initially headquartered in San Diego, it decided that the greener pastures of the District of Columbia were a better move in 1985. In 1988, another activity of the group was that

> Escuela de la Libertad (School of Liberty) was built and sponsored by CWA in the jungle of Costa Rica for Nicaraguan refugee children. Meanwhile, CWA's open-air medical clinics at the school offered physical, emotional and spiritual assistance.[29]

In 1991, CWA became interested in the RU-486 project, becoming active with the NRLC in meeting "with European companies engaged in the production of RU-486." CWA was one of the few pro-life groups to voice public disagreement with Texas governor Rick Perry's 2007 Gardasil mandate. In the 1990s, CWA was mindful of increasing its public profile and weighed in against stem-cell research and Plan B.

The histories of the FRC and FOF are discussed together since they tried to work as one organization from 1988 to 1992. FOF was first on the radar screen, according to its website, when Dr. James Dobson began broadcasting his family-based radio show in 1977. Like the LaHayes, Dobson began his organization in California (Arcadia), later moving to Colorado Springs, Colorado, its present-day home.[30] In 1980, while the LaHayes were holding an alternative conference to the White House Family Conference as the co-chairs designated by the National Pro-Family Coalition, Dobson was invited to participate in the 1980 White House Conference on Families, according to his organization's website.

The competition for policy space inside the pro-life/pro-family movement has been keen since the 1970s. In another development related to the expansion of one's territory, FOF had an office in Canada as early as 1984; it set up another lobbying office in Ottawa, the capital, in 2006 at the time of the federal election when the Conservatives were elected. As with the Rockefeller Foundation and the Population Council, FOF seems to have become one of the nexus points for the pro-life side's money. For example, the network of crisis pregnancy centers, CARENET and Birthright, mention significant donations from FOF. FOF, like many other groups in the pro-choice and pro-life constellations, has been putting up its recent federal tax returns on its website. The numbers show that it is in a similar realm to PPFA. While PPFA showed 89 million dollars in assets in 2007, FOF listed 96 million dollars.[31]

The FRC was founded under the following circumstances. According to its website, www.frc.org,

> After attending a research planning meeting for President Carter's 1980 White House Conference on Families, Dr. James Dobson met and prayed with a group of eight Christian leaders at a Washington hotel. From that beginning resolve was formed to establish the Family Research Council, and one of those present that night, Gerald P. Regier, became our first president. FRC's immediate goal was to counter the credentialed voices arrayed against life and family with equally capable men and women of faith.[32]

By 1988, the FRC had joined FOF and was then headed by Gary Bauer, domestic policy advisor to President Reagan and former undersecretary of education.[33]

The marriage between FOF and the FRC was short-lived, when FRC broke away to have its own board and director. It set up its own building, funded by the Prince and DeVos families of Michigan. Erik Prince, heir to the family fortune, has worked at both FRC and FOF. His sister is married into the DeVos family, and his mother, Elsa, has also sat on both FRC and FOF boards. He is a major donor to conservative, pro-life members of Congress, including former Representative and now Senator (and MD) Tom Coburn. Coburn was one of the House leaders in the fight against RU-486 importation and one of the initiators of the Title V Social Security Act in 1996, authorizing funding for abstinence-only education programs, including anti-choice crisis pregnancy centers.[34] Prince is probably most famous for being the founder and CEO of the mercenary security firm, Blackwater Worldwide. The DeVos family, like the Van Andel one, is one of the controlling interests in Amway. The FRC website says that in addition to the DC office, a distribution center was founded in Holland, Michigan. That area is in social conservative territory, with a strong following in the Calvinist Dutch Reform Church, claiming members of the DeVos, VanAndel, and Prince families. One wonders exactly what is being distributed at the distribution center; the FRC website is silent on that.

Other foundations that have been identified as strong supporters of the New Right include those of Mellon, DeMoss, Bradley, Scaife, Kirby, Earhart, Hume, Castle Rock, Coors, and Smith Richardson, among others.[35] If one were to visit the Heritage Foundation in Washington, DC, one would find the names of the Scaife and Coors foundations emblazoned in an archway over the door.[36]

Other active groups in the pro-life coalition groups are Physicians for Life, Nurses for Life, and Pharmacists for Life. The website of the former states, interestingly, that its Canadian side was formed in 1975 (much earlier than in the United States), with the U.S. group starting in 1986 as an Alabama chapter and the national organization starting at an unspecified date thereafter.[37] Pharmacists for Life International (PFLI) states on its website that it was founded in 1984 in Ohio. It also states:

> PFLI is a worldwide apostolate of thousands of pharmacists, plus hundreds of other health professionals, pharmacy students, interns, pharmacy technicians, and the public, in the USA, Canada and worldwide. We are represented on all of the continents except Antarctica, with active regional coordinators in many states and nations.[38]

The groups Physicians for Life, Nurses for Life, and Pharmacists for Life participate in blocking women's access to services at the provision point. In most cases, they violate statutory or constitutional law that has established women's rights to access this type of care. In Canada, the same landscape holds true except that the hospitals and clinics, not the provinces, are the levels at which the refusal policies are adopted and implemented.[39] While Physicians for Life and Nurses for Life are often found in Catholic-owned hospitals, which comprise 12 percent each of the U.S. and Canadian landscapes, their members can claim exemption from providing services in any public or private hospital subject to the policy.[40] A significant problem in both the United States and Canada is that virtually no accountability mechanisms are in place to stop the manipulation of these policies by anti-choice providers. For example, doctors and nurses will routinely not pass on the names of pro-choice providers or clinics as most conscience clauses require. Other frontline violators of women's rights include those answering the telephones at clinics or hospitals who falsely claim ignorance of a venue's pro-choice policy or incorrectly describe it as anti-choice only.[41] For many years, pharmacists in the United States and Canada violated the alternatives embedded in the conscience clause policy that was to inform clients where or when a pro-choice pharmacist would be available. The pharmacy issue has been onerous with regard to Plan B in both the United States and Canada.[42]

A seemingly contradictory strategy has been pursued by the New Right since the 1980s. The first has been to pay strong attention to building an infrastructure at the state level. This structure includes a web of mini–Heritage Foundations and mini-FRCs, to solidify the policy presence of the right.[43] This infrastructure has come in particularly handy as state legislators have crafted conservative legislation and conservative lawyers have contested against pro-choice laws in the states. On the other hand, the federal level has also been targeted by the New Right, and in particular, the Department of Health and Human Services (HHS) due to its presence in administering the bulk of family-related program money in the United States.

In terms of establishing the state-level think-tank networks, a key player is said to be Don Eberly of Pennsylvania, a cofounder with Wade Horn of the National Fatherhood Initiative in 1994.[44] According to Clarkson, the goals behind the conservative think-tank infrastructure build have been not only to act as liaisons and funders to candidates but also to state Republican parties as strategists and mentors, to "take the Reagan revolution to the states," and to groom federal candidates.[45] Clarkson notes that the mini-Heritage idea was broached at a 1986 conference at the Madison Hotel in Washington, DC, and the idea for the network was originally to call it the Madison Group. In 1992, it was renamed the State Policy Network (SPN) and in 1999 was said to have 37 organizations in 30 different states. This network represents mainly financial conservative interests.[46] Social conservative interests are represented through the network of family policy councils, started in 1988 under James Dobson and FOE[47] In 1999, there were 34 of these state-based groups. Dobson also funded the Promise Keepers, the report stated. The family policy councils usually work more on social issues, but at times will combine with SPNs to reach more voters or legislators, whomever the target is. As conservative farm teams at the state levels, the two networks hire former Congressional aides and also former employees have been elected as governors and state legislators.[48] As with the groups Physicians for Life et al., concerted attention has been paid to enacting robust networks to change policy on the front lines, whether it be in a hospital or in a state legislature.

The federal level of social conservative strategies was continued from the Hatch and Hyde Amendments of the 1970s into the 1980s. Social conservatives in Congress quickly started to challenge public funding for contraception. As noted by Alesha Doan and Jean Williams, the beginning of abstinence-based education in 1980 by Senators Jeremiah Denton and Orrin Hatch was "expressly for the purpose of diverting (federal) money that would otherwise go to Planned Parenthood to groups with traditional values."[49] Specifically, the Adolescent Family Life Act (AFLA) was added as Title XX of the Public Health Service Act, to counteract Title X that had been added in 1970 to publicly fund contraception. AFLA also set up the Office of Adolescent Pregnancy Prevention within the newly created HHS. According to Rebekah Saul of the Guttmacher Institute, AFLA was intended to stop mainly teenage sexual activity and to encourage adoption over abortion.[50] The program devoted two-thirds of its funding to the care of pregnant teenagers and one-third of the funding to prevention efforts. These percentages were reversed in the 1996 welfare reform legislation, the

Personal Responsibility and Opportunity Work Reconciliation Act. Another part of the legislation predating the Reagan administration's 1984 Mexico City policy was to refuse to provide any funding for groups (such as IPPF) advocating abortion.

Social conservatives were even bolder after the second major step of the rolling Republican realignment in 1994 with the historic win of both houses of Congress, a majority of the nation's governorships (giving Republicans large amounts of state-level veto power), and the rise of Speaker Gingrich. The House in particular turned sharply to the right, with many more social conservatives, including the speaker, in leadership and the rank and file. The next iteration of abstinence-based programming was much broader in scope and implementation powers than AFLA had been. It was passed in the same manner as AFLA, as an amendment to the fiscal year 1997 budget reconciliation process by Speaker Gingrich. The speaker's action was taken at the behest of two conservative Oklahoma members, Representatives Tom Coburn and Ernest Istook.[51]

As noted by Saul and by Doan and Williams, the 1996 legislation was intended to discourage promiscuity (sex outside marriage), irrespective of a woman's age. It also awarded 250 million dollars for 5 years to the program, administered through the Maternal and Child Health Bureau, established as part of Title V of the Social Security Act of 1935. In 1981, Title V had been changed to a block-grant program, and the abstinence-based only provision was Section 510 of Title V.[52] In 1991, the Administration on Children, Youth and Families (ACYF) was created by President George H. W. Bush. Recipients of Title V funding could only promote abstinence and marriage but not contraception.

A prominent actor in the conversion mechanism of ACYF was Wade Horn, head of the conservative Fatherhood Initiative, commissioner of the ACYF, and chief of the Children's Bureau at HHS during the George H. W. Bush presidency, from 1989 to 1993. From 2001 to 2007, Horn served as assistant secretary of the ACYF for President George W. Bush and as assistant secretary for Community Initiatives in HHS as well. At least one of his actions in converting the ACYF and Title V involved giving 12 million dollars to his former organization, the National Fatherhood Initiative, in a no-bid, 5-year contract. Horn was identified as George W. Bush's point man on abstinence-based funding, welfare reform (Personal Responsibility and Work Opportunity Reconciliation Act), and Head Start.[53]

CONCLUSION

Most elements of institutional theory, historical and discursive, have been shown to be applicable in this chapter. First, clear discursive shifts from the first policy punctuation to the second are evident. While the passage of Title X in 1970 was not directly tied to a massive lobbying effort on the part of women, it is clear that *Roe v. Wade* was the outcome of lobbying by doctors, lawyers, and women who wanted a new framework on abortion policy. Thus, the discursive framework of the first policy period was shared by explicitly feminist groups such as NARAL and also the older demography-related groups such as the Rockefeller Foundation. The discursive framework of the second policy period was reminiscent of the Comstock era, in which anti-choice organizations hewed to a traditional view of the family and of women's roles in it. Pro-choice organizations worked hard to counter this view through the use of public discourse, but by 1980 the state institutions had become more representative of conservative viewpoints than liberal ones.

During the Clinton administrations of 1992–2000, pro-choice organizations worked to layer in feminist understandings of women's reproductive autonomy, especially around the issues of medical abortion, emergency contraception, and abstinence-based education. The layering concept of historical institutionalism is helpful in this regard because while the Clinton administration ultimately was helpful with the combination of emergency contraception and RU-486, it was less so with regard to Plan B. President Clinton also supported welfare reform and thus did not work to counteract the massive abstinence-based groundwork laid by members of Congress, which became a super-structure during the George W. Bush presidencies.

While the changes found in the first policy system were embedded in the health policy network through layering onto existing ones, those of the second policy system were clearly due to outright conversion from progressive understandings of women's roles to conservative ones. The conversion of funding mechanisms for contraception also involved policy drift since fewer women needing access to contraceptive and abortion services were eligible to receive public funding.[54] Other examples of conversion involved passage of Title XX of the Public Health Service Act to counteract Title X and the conversion of Title V of the Social Security Act of 1935 to conservative ends.

While feminist and pro-choice organizations had flourished nationally in the 1970s, the cusp of the policy punctuation on women's reproductive rights, they were consistently put in a reactive position in the 1980s and sometimes in the 1990s. This location was in part due to the conservative movement's success in establishing a wide-ranging network at the state level to constantly challenge previous laws and implement new anti-choice ones.

NOTES

1. Walter Dean Burnham, *Critical Elections: And the Mainsprings of American Politics* (New York: W. W. Norton & Company, 1971) and James L. Sundquist, *Dynamics of the*

Party System: The Growth and Realignment of Political Parties in the US, revised ed. (Washington, DC: Brookings, 1983).

2. Clare Coleman and Kirtly Parker, M.D., "Title X: A Proud Past, an Uncertain Future," *Contraception* 84, no. 3 (2011): 209–11.

3. Ibid.

4. Patricia Sullivan, Obituary on Lawrence Lader, *Washington Post*, May 11, 2006, B6.

5. Melissa Haussman, *Abortion Politics in North America* (Boulder, CO: Lynne Rienner, 2005), 29.

6. "History and Successes" *Planned Parenthood*, http://www.plannedparenthood.org/about-us/who-we-are/history-and-successes.htm?__utma=1.368788854.1342294630.1342294630.1342294630.1342294630.1&__utmb=1.6.10.1342294630&__utmc=1&__utmx=-&__utmz=1.1342294630.1.1.utmcsr=(direct)|utmccn=(direct)|utmcmd=(none)&__utmv=-&__utmk=126293517.

7. Ibid.

8. Donald Critchlow, *Intended Consequences: Birth Control, Abortion and the Modern American Government* (New York: Oxford University Press, 1999), Chapters 2 and 4.

9. *PATH*, www.path.org.

10. "The Birth of Path," *PATH*, http://www.path.org/about/birth-of-path.php.

11. Patricia Sellers, "Melinda Gates Goes Public," *CNN Money*, January 7, 2008, http://money.cnn.com/2008/01/04/news/newsmakers/gates.fortune/index.htm.

12. "Initiatives on Public-Private Partnerships for Health," *Concept Foundation*, March 7, 2006, http://www.conceptfoundation.org.

13. "Realizing the Mission-Managing the Evolution," *Concept Foundation*, http://www.conceptfoundation.org.

14. *Guttmacher Institute*, www.guttmacher.org.

15. *Center for Reproductive Rights*, www.reproductiverights.org.

16. Ibid.

17. William Saletan, *Bearing Right: How Conservatives Won the Abortion War* (Berkeley, CA: University of California Press, 2004), 257.

18. Ibid., 231.

19. Ibid.

20. Critchlow, *Intended Consequences*, Chapters 2 and 4.

21. Wolfgang Streeck and Kathleen Thelen, eds., *Beyond Continuity: Institutional Change in Advanced Political Economies* (London: Oxford University Press, 2005), 1–39 and Jacob S. Hacker, "Policy Drift: The Hidden Politics of US Welfare State Retrenchment," in Streeck and Thelen, *Beyond Continuity*, 40–83.

22. Coleman and Parker, "Title X," 209–11.

23. *National Right to Life Committee*, www.nrlc.org.

24. *Americans United for Life*, www.aul.org.

25. *American Life League*, www.all.org.

26. "State Policies in Brief: Refusal Clauses," *Guttmacher Institute*, http://www.guttmacher.org/statecenter/spibs/spib_RPHS.pdf.

27. "State Policies in Brief: Public Funding for Abortion," *Guttmacher Institute*, http://www.guttmacher.org/statecenter/spibs/spib_SFAM.pdf.

28. "Our History," *Concerned Women for America*, http://www.cwfa.org/about.asp.

29. *Concerned Women for America*, http://www.cwfa.org/main.asp.

30. "Historical Timeline," *Focus on the Family*, http://www.focusonthefamily.com/about_us/news_room/history.aspx.

31. "Financial Reports," *Focus on the Family*, http://www.focusonthefamily.com/about_us/financial_reports.aspx.

32. *Family Research Council*, www.frc.org.

33. Ibid.

34. "Erik Prince," *Right Web*, http://rightweb.irc-online.org/profile/Prince_Erik/.

35. Liz Hrenda-Roberts, "Money, Power and the Radical Right in Pennsylvania," *PADNET*, http://www.padnet.org/mprrcont.html.

36. As this author did when accompanying a group of university students to Washington, DC, in 2003.

37. *Physicians for Life*, www.physiciansforlife.org.

38. *Pharmacists for Life International*, www.pfli.org.

39. "The Canadian Abortion Provider Shortage: Now and Tomorrow," *Abortion Rights Coalition of Canada*, Position Paper No. 5, October 2005, http://arcc-cdac.ca/postionpapers/05-Abortion-Provider-Shortage.PDF.

40. Ibid. and Jerry Filteau, "Catholic Hospitals Serve One in Six Patients in the US," *National Catholic Reporter*, October 20, 2010, http://ncronline.org/news/catholic-hospitals-serve-one-six-patients-united-states.

41. Jessica Shaw, "Reality Check: A Close Look at Accessing Abortion Services in Canadian Hospitals," *Canadians for Choice*, April 2, 2007, http://www.canadiansforchoice.ca/reportspeech.pdf and Melissa Haussman and Pauline Rankin, "Framing the Harper Government: Gender-Neutral during Elections while Gender-Negative in Caucus," in *How Ottawa Spends, 2009–2010*, ed. Allan Maslove (Montreal: McGill-Queen's Press, 2009), Chapter 10.

42. Ibid.

43. Frederick Clarkson, "Takin' It to the States: The Rise of Conservative State-Level Think Tanks," *The Public Eye*, XIII, nos. 2–3 (Summer/Fall 1999), http://www.publiceye.org/magazine/v13n2-3/PE_V13_N2-3.pdf.

44. Hrenda-Roberts, "Money, Power and the Radical Right in Pennsylvania."

45. Clarkson, "Takin' It to the States."

46. Ibid.

47. Ibid.

48. Ibid.

49. Alesha E. Doan and Jean Calterone Williams, *The Politics of Virginity: Abstinence in Sex Education* (Westport, CT: Praeger, 2008), 28 and Susan Rose, "Going Too Far? Sex, Sin and Social Policy," *Social Forces* 84, no. 2 (December 2005): 1207–32.

50. Rebekah Saul, "Whatever Happened to the Adolescent Family Life Act?" *Guttmacher Report on Public Policy* 1, no. 2 (April 1998), http://www.guttmacher.org/pubs/tgr/01/2/gr010205.html.

51. Doan and Williams, *The Politics of Virginity*, 33.

52. *Maternal and Child Health Bureau,* http://mchb.hrsa.gov/.

53. Bill Berkowitz, "Wade Horn Cashes Out," *Media Transparency,* April 25, 2007, http://abatteredmother.wordpress.com/2011/04/14/wade-horn-cashes-out/.

54. Streeck and Thelen, *Beyond Continuity*, 1–39.

5

Problems with Mifepristone (RU–486) and Misoprostol (Cytotec), 1988–2000

This chapter's focus is on RU-486, the mifepristone pill, developed in France in 1980 and kept off the U.S. market by a combination of economic protectionist and social conservative interests until 2000. The fight over RU-486 is firmly lodged in the second policy period on women's reproductive drugs and rights.

This chapter continues the central two arguments of the book with regard to this case study. The first argument is that the for-profit nature of the U.S.-based pharma industry is central to explaining the choices made by the public and private sectors. The second argument is that the drug policymaking process in the United States is fundamentally gendered since women have not yet been included as equal participants. Women are treated by the pharma giants as clients of the system, whose interests can be ignored or postponed. Starting with the RU-486 example, though, it is possible to see evidence of prominent women MD's and researchers forming companies to help with Food and Drug Administration (FDA) approval or marketing of the product, either in the U.S. or global system.

RELEVANT U.S. DRUGS IN EXISTENCE PRIOR
TO RU-486 (METHOTREXATE AND MISOPROSTOL)

In pharma politics, the story centers just as much on the fortunes (real or perceived) of a specific company as it does the specific drug under discussion. What is interesting about the case of mifepristone (RU-486) is that it was not kept out of the United States due to observed safety or efficacy concerns, since it did precisely what it was supposed to do, that is expel the contents of the uterus. Presidents Reagan and George H. W. Bush, and therefore the FDA, kept it out of the country under spurious safety concerns although similar drugs had been in the United States for years. Methotrexate was approved as an anti-cancer drug by the FDA in 1961, and the FDA allowed misoprostol to be marketed for gastric ulcers, starting in 1988. Methotrexate, patented by Lederle, a division of the U.S. company Wyeth Labs, is an anti-folic acid receptor and was first tested in the 1940s. It quickly became the number one anti-cancer drug in the United States for decades, thus it was a blockbuster. It was soon discovered to be effective at inducing labor in women, and thus medical (nonsurgical or chemical) abortion. It has been one of the (off-label) drugs for choice in treating ectopic pregnancies.[1]

Misoprostol, a prostaglandin patented by Searle in 1976 and sold as Cytotec, was approved by the FDA in 1988 although it had been studied and used in trials since the 1970s. Notably, methotrexate and misoprostol can be used alone or together to induce cervical thinning and uterine contractions for either abortion or birth. Given misoprostol's (Cytotec's) effectiveness in reproductive and gynecological matters, it was routinely used off-label. It has also been used to stop postpartum hemorrhaging. Misoprostol has been viewed by the medical community as a good drug in various settings and frequently has been used off-label in Latin America and East Asia. It is a highly stable compound requiring no refrigeration.[2] For inducing labor, misoprostol is faster than Pitocin, which is administered through an IV drip. Thus, time-pressed doctors liked misoprostol as it fit with their own schedules. Cytotec can bring on such strong contractions that it ruptures the uterus and thus women need to be within close range of medical follow-up. One estimate was that 150,000 doctors were using Cytotec off-label to induce labor by the early 1990s.[3] While misoprostol (Cytotec) can be used alone for a medical abortion, the success rate goes up to 92 percent when used in combination with mifepristone (RU-486) during the first 7 weeks of pregnancy. Similarly, studies showed that mifepristone alone was only effective 60–80 percent of the time in performing a complete medical abortion, but when combined with misoprostol, the rates were increased to 95 percent effectiveness. The mifepristone regimen must be used within seven weeks of the last missed period in order to work, since later in pregnancy mifepristone cannot sufficiently block out the placenta's natural hormones.[4]

The big difference with RU-486 (mifepristone) is that medical abortion was its chief function, although given the similarities to the other two drugs it could be used for the treatment of Cushing's disease, a condition indicated by high levels of cortisone steroids in the body, or cancer. Mifepristone, a progestin (i.e., synthesized hormone), works as a glucocorticoid/progesterone receptor antagonist. Mifepristone causes the placenta to separate from the uterine lining, softens the cervix, and increases uterine contractions. A medical abortion conducted with three tablets, 200 milligrams each of the anti-progestational drug mifepristone (which works to thin the uterine lining) typically needs to be followed two days later with 0.4 grams (400 micrograms) of misoprostol (two tablets) to make sure the abortion is complete.

The owner of the Cytotec patent, the Searle company, consistently lobbied against having its drug included in an official medical-abortion procedure. The company also claimed that it did not want the drug used for labor purposes in delivery rooms since the pill did not warrant enough revenue for the perceived risks to the company.[5] In August 2000, one month after the drug had gone off-patent, Searle sent a letter to medical practitioners to warn them that Cytotec was not FDA-approved for labor or abortion induction, although practitioners already knew that.[6] It has strongly been suggested that the timing of that action was linked to avoiding future liability. Until misoprostol went off-patent in July 2000, Searle acted to push any potential U.S. manufacturer away from making mifepristone, since misoprostol would be required as an accompaniment.

In addition to its earlier history of foot-dragging on the contraceptive pill's research in the United States, Searle's later behavior is relevant to the RU-486 story. Searle was bought by Monsanto in 1985, after Donald Rumsfeld had chaired the company from 1977 to 1985, closing divisions and firing a quarter of its workforce to make the company more profitable and attractive for a takeover. From the perspective of Monsanto, buying Searle and making it a wholly-owned subsidiary was said to end its long efforts to associate itself with an experienced pharma company with an ethical reputation.[7] As an agribusiness company, Monsanto had had its share of controversy, as it and Merrell-Dow were the largest sellers of the defoliant Agent Orange. Monsanto has been the largest developer of genetically modified agricultural products, and was a major producer of polychlorinated biphenyls (PCBs, which are industrial chemicals). In addition to cancers, birth defects and nervous system damage produced by Agent Orange and PCB, other Monsanto products such as DDT and Roundup have been similarly implicated. Just after Monsanto purchased Searle, it learned that Searle was facing more than 300 lawsuits for millions of dollars over its Copper 7 IUD (intrauterine device). The

IUD had been wrongly marketed by Searle primarily to young women who had never been pregnant, and caused numerous health problems including pelvic infections, ectopic pregnancies, and infertility. After losing a jury trial with a judgment of 8.75 million dollars in 1988 and its liability insurance coverage for the product, Searle settled the other lawsuits. It withdrew the Copper 7 from the market in 1986.[8]

Rumsfeld's pugnaciousness as Searle's head has been noted. When Searle was having difficulty in getting aspartame, its artificial sweetener, through the FDA approvals process, Rumsfeld claimed in 1981 that he could force aspartame through the process based not on the science, but on his political connections. As a member of Ronald Reagan's transition team, Rumsfeld helped pick a business (and Searle)-friendly FDA commissioner, Dr. Arthur Hayes, who stacked an FDA committee in favor of the aspartame decision well within the 1981 time frame promised by Rumsfeld. In addition, relevant to the Plan B circumstances, Hayes overruled the FDA committee that advised against allowing aspartame for use in dry products.[9] Monsanto was sold to Pharmacia in 1999 (a Swedish-based firm, founded in 1911). Pharmacia had previously merged with Upjohn, and the Pharmacia–Upjohn–Monsanto merger became Pharmacia in 2000. In 1995, Searle acquired the Swiss Roche company's Syntex holdings, thus buying out its former birth-control pill competitor from the 1950s. Pfizer bought Pharmacia (and discontinued the Searle brand) in 2003. With these acquisitions, Pfizer became the world's largest pharma company and the largest owner of oral contraceptive patents.

RU-486 was first formulated in France by the Roussel Uclaf company in 1980 and licensed in 1982. It also was copied (illegally, off-patent) by the Chinese in the early 1980s, who licensed a mifepristone-based pill in 1988 to help enforce the one-child policy. A majority share of Roussel Uclaf had been sold to the German company Hoechst in 1994 (the rest of the shares were purchased by Hoechst in 1997).

Originally, Roussel Uclaf, the manufacturer of RU-486, worked with the U.S.-based Population Council to test the drug. It was tested as an anti-cancer drug beginning in 1983 at the University of Southern California (USC) and later at the National Institutes of Health (NIH), but specifically as an abortifacient in studies conducted jointly by the NIH, the Population Council, and USC Medical School from 1983 to 1987. Interestingly, RU-486 had not yet been officially licensed in either France or the United States at the time. The second wave was a 17-site trial conducted by the Population Council, begun in 1994. It was also announced that year by the Marie Stopes Clinics in Britain that they would provide mifepristone to U.S. women who flew there to get it.[10] Roussel Uclaf (and its parent company Hoechst) consistently displayed nervousness about bringing the drug to the United States. In 1989, it forced the trials in California to be halted.[11]

THE BUSINESS AND SOCIAL CONSERVATIVE LOBBY AGAINST RU-486

The American Legislative Exchange Council (ALEC) was formed in 1973 to give social and economic conservatives and corporations a direct role in policy-making, different from physical lobbying of legislators. ALEC's purpose is drafting model legislation usually for the state level but sometimes targeted at the federal level. One example was a 1996 model bill written at the behest of pharma companies represented by ALEC to decrease wait times for drug approval at the FDA.[12] The council's website describes itself as "a nonpartisan membership association for conservative state lawmakers who share (d) a belief in limited government, free markets, federalism and individual liberty."[13] Instrumental early adherents and founders included then State Representative Henry Hyde, Tommy Thompson of Wisconsin (George W. Bush's secretary of HHS and overseer of the FDA during his first term), and Senator Jesse Helms. Clearly, Helms and Hyde learned a lot from their association with ALEC in terms of making federal legislation more conservative-friendly.

Wendell Potter, a former insurance industry executive, wrote about ALEC in *The Nation* in August 2011, showing ALEC's work to cut back federal health insurance benefits and to increase the role of private corporations in health service delivery, including in Medicare and Medicaid. The latter is also a proposal by current Budget chair and Tea-Party member Representative Paul Ryan.[14] One of ALEC's proposals that has become law in three states concerned the availability of private health-insurance schemes. These laws created insurance pools that cross state lines, which is ironic given the conservative antipathy for the Obama administration's Patient Protection and Affordable Care Act (PPACA) requirement of mandating state insurance coverage. Unlike the ALEC laws that cut benefits by making the insurance pools larger, the PPACA seeks to improve insurance coverage, and of course that is what the industry opposes. As Potter summed up, ALEC's goals against Obama's health-care law, largely realized, were "a well-coordinated effort to keep the most progressive proposals from being enacted at the state or federal level." It was not successful in killing the provisions to increase insurance industry business oversight.[15]

Corporations that are represented on ALEC's board and are relevant to this study include Pfizer, Bayer (a representative of which co-chaired the ALEC Task Force on Health and Pharmaceuticals), Johnson & Johnson, and GlaxoSmith-Kline. Not surprisingly, the largest global corporation Walmart is a member. Donald Rumsfeld was a member of the Business Policy Task Force in 1983, while he was chair of Searle in 1977–1985 and of the task force in 1995.

The ALEC website also states that the association started seven issue-area task forces in response to President Reagan's 1981 Task Force on Federalism. These were later called Cabinet Task Forces, and ALEC claims that the Presidential Task Force relied heavily on ALEC members for testimony, and that the groups worked directly with the administration on key issues.[16] The ALEC site also states that

> In 1982, ALEC began developing its first health care initiatives. After much success with policy formation and education, in 1986, ALEC made a commitment to form formal internal Task Forces to develop policy covering virtually every responsibility of state government . . . the Health Care Task Force had developed policies on medical savings accounts, a concerted strategy for reassessing mandated coverage, and a comprehensive response to the growing AIDS crisis.[17]

ALEC's work with the Presidential Task Force on Federalism is consistent with conservatives' emphasis on state-level infrastructure creation described by Clarkson.[18] This scenario has been fulfilled, whereby the firms, think tanks, and task forces exist to support conservative state legislators in framing policy and lawyers in challenging progressive policies.

A major nongovernmental-organization player in the New Right anti-contraception and abortion battle since the second half of the 20th century has been the U.S. National Right to Life Committee (NRLC). One of the prominent founders was physician John Wilke. In 1987, he founded the International Right to Life Committee, with chapters conveniently located in both France where Roussel Uclaf was headquartered and in Italy where the Vatican is based. Early tactics against RU-486 and its parent company Hoechst included three prongs: warnings that they would embarrass the company internationally, work to bankrupt it, and go after any companies holding stock in Hoechst or RU-486. One key strategy was to identify Hoechst, the owner of Roussel Uclaf, as itself a founding member of (and then spun-off component of) I. G. Farben company. Farben—once the fourth-largest company in the world after General Motors, Standard Oil, and U.S. Steel—was comprised in 1925 as a conglomerate of eight different companies, of which Hoechst and Bayer were two of the largest. In 1951, the Western allies divided up the company after the Soviets had appropriated assets in the Eastern Bloc. Two of the largest original Farben components remained under the names of Bayer and Hoechst; Farben still exists on paper as a company. The strategy of the NRLC was to publicly tie Hoechst-Roussel to Farben as the patent holder of Zyklon B.[19]

In 1988, the NRLC helped to form a lobby group that then registered with Congress, named after the Robins-Carbide-Reynolds company, RCR Alliance. These companies had all suffered large liability claims and the RCR Alliance existed "solely to pressure Roussel Uclaf and Hoechst not to license RU-486 and not to provide it to other countries."[20] The fact that Hoechst had a U.S. base in New Jersey also made it open to pressure by the NRLC and its allies, and also the fact that the German head of Hoechst was Catholic ultimately played a large role in Hoechst's stated unwillingness to pursue FDA approval. Julie Hogan has written that part of the RCR Alliance's tactics was to threaten that it would find plaintiffs in developing countries where RU-486 might be distributed.[21]

What is ironic about the companies with ties to Farben (Bayer and Hoechst directly, Monsanto through a joint venture) is that none of these companies were angels in practice or theory. Farben held the patent for Zyklon B and Monsanto has produced some of the most noxious chemicals used on the globe. However, Searle under Monsanto refused to tie itself to an official protocol for medical abortion. Its influence was felt in that according to Hogan, Schering-Plough, Johnson & Johnson, Pharmacia, Upjohn, and Pfizer, all refused to become the U.S. manufacturer for mifepristone.[22] The last three companies were all tied directly to Monsanto, sequentially buying each other out. Pharmacia and Monsanto were said to share the same headquarters and personnel even when they were supposedly separate legal entities.[23] Thus, these companies were open to pressure by Searle and Monsanto against getting involved in the RU-486 and misoprostol fights. Some of the five also worked with Searle in ALEC. Other companies—including Teva (the world's leading generics company and the current producer of Plan B in 2012), Merck (which produces Gardasil), Abbott Laboratories, and Johnson & Johnson—were "lobbied vigorously by conservative investment funds" and thus declined to participate.[24] It is thus clear that no matter what unseemly drugs these companies had previously produced, they portrayed themselves as squeezed on one side by Hoechst-Roussel and the NRLC's war against it and Searle's insistence on keeping misoprostol (Cytotec) out of a medical-abortion regime at least until its patent ran out in July 2000.

THE 1988–1989 IMPORT ALERT ON MIFEPRISTONE (RU-486)

In July 1988, the FDA was directed to revise its procedures on drugs that did not yet have U.S.-based trial results and thus had not been approved by the FDA. This procedure was to allow small amounts of such drugs (originally for cancer or HIV/AIDS treatments) into the United States via the mail.[25] Forty drugs were listed as being outside the purview of the exemption, and in November 1988, the FDA declared that RU-486 was not on the banned list. The need for the 1988 changes is unclear, since the stated policy in effect since 1977 was that "the FDA will not detain unapproved new drugs imported for personal use."[26] In February 1989, the

FDA revised its Regulatory Procedures Manual to effect the changes, framed again as the Personal Use Exemption, under which importation for personal use of any drug not listed in an import alert was subject to a case-by-case discretionary decision by the FDA.[27] The FDA laid out several decision-making criteria:

> When the intended use is appropriately identified, such use is not for treatment of a serious condition, and the product is not known to represent a significant health risk; or when (1) the intended use is unapproved and for a serious condition for which effective treatment may not be available domestically, either through commercial or clinical means; (2) there is no known commercialization or promotion to persons residing in the United States . . . ; (3) the product is considered not to represent an unreasonable risk; and (4) the individual seeking to import the product affirms in writing that it is for the patient's own personal use . . . RPM 9-71-30(C).[28]

On May 5, 1989, three anti-choice House members (Conservatives Robert Dornan of California, Henry Hyde of Illinois, and John LaFalce of New York, the only Democrat among these three) wrote to Commissioner Frank Young of the FDA, a Reagan appointee. Their complaint was that the FDA had not included RU-486 on the list of 40 drugs banned from the personal exemption procedure and therefore could still be imported. Senator Jesse Helms followed up shortly thereafter. Soon after Helms's letter to Commissioner Young, the FDA violated its own procedure by putting in an addendum to the Regulatory Procedures Manual to ban RU-486 for import to the public, but not to doctors. Since a public notice to this effect was not published in the *Federal Register* before the change was added to the Regulatory Procedures Manual, legal analysts have stated that the FDA violated Section 553 of the Administrative Procedures Act. That section requires public comment periods after publication of the proposed change. That was not followed in this case.[29] Similarly, while Carpenter believes that FDA policy cannot be inferred from a presidential stance, it is clear that Commissioner Young was following the expressed desire of President George H.W. Bush, mainly to get rid of RU-486 as a political target. Similarly, this action gave breathing room to Searle until Cytotec went off-patent in 2000. Thus, Searle did not have to publicly defend itself against a public push for RU-486, which required Cytotect (misoprostol) to be effective.[30]

The FDA's addition of RU-486 to the list of drugs that could not be imported for personal use came in the form of FDA Import Alert 66-47, issued on June 6, 1989. The import alert's language was modeled directly on the surviving aspect of the Comstock Law, which "directs customs officials to automatically detain all shipments of unapproved abortifacient drugs."[31] While the language from 1977 of the Regulatory Procedures Manual had stated that "the FDA will not prevent unapproved drugs from entering the US for personal use," the import alert shifted the burden to the Customs Service. The 1989 alert was somewhat less severe than the Comstock legislation had been on abortifacients since the alert at least allowed physicians to keep receiving RU-486, and individuals simply could not import it for their own purposes. As Chicoine notes, though, the effect of the alert was to basically halt clinical trials on RU-486 at the time.[32] Another related measure was that Congressman Tom Coburn of Oklahoma attached riders to the agriculture budgets in 1998 and 2000 (which were dropped) to prohibit RU-486 research funding. The import alert on RU-486 was not rescinded until fall 2000, just before the Clinton administration left office.

As Margaret Sanger had tested the Comstock Act prohibitions against importing contraceptives through the mail to U.S. doctors and won in the *One Package* decisions of 1936, so too did journalist and longtime pro-choice activist Lawrence Lader test the constitutionality of the FDA Import Alert of June 1989 regarding RU-486. Lader was a longtime pro-choice activist and a follower and biographer of Margaret Sanger's. Lader writes that he borrowed the idea for a court challenge directly from Sanger's 1934 actions. In 1992, he searched for the perfect plaintiff, a healthy, nonsmoking woman less than seven weeks pregnant. RU-486 is not effective seven weeks after a woman's last missed period. Pro-choice activist Leona Benten volunteered and in late June 1992, she and Lader flew to Britain to get the dosages of RU-486 and misoprostol from an unnamed doctor. Following Sanger's procedures 60 years earlier, Lader alerted the customs officials and the press as to his intentions while the trip was in progress. Thus, when Lader and Benten arrived in New York on July 1, 1992, their names were registered at Customs, and Ms. Benten was taken aside. Lader was carrying the misoprostol, which was illegal since he did not have a prescription for it in the United States, and Benten was carrying the RU-486 (mifepristone), which was also clearly illegal. U.S. Customs seized both sets of pills.[33] The sought-after media attention was present, and the Center for Reproductive Law and Policy (CRLP) phoned to offer its pro-bono services as Lader and Benten prepared a lawsuit against the U.S. Customs Service. The central claim of the lawsuit was that adding RU-486 to the Import Alert violated a previous 1977 rule, the personal exemption, whereby small quantities of unapproved drugs could be imported for personal use if a similar substitute were not available in the United States. Since a substitute was not available, Lader and Benten's actions were aimed at getting the Import Alert against RU-486 overturned. Lader stated that the government attorneys defending the alert "insisted that the personal-use exemption applied only to illnesses like Parkinson's and AIDS . . . they were thus placing pregnant women in an inferior category."[34]

On July 14, 1992, Brooklyn federal district court Judge Charles Sifton, a Carter appointee, termed the scenario "a lawsuit waiting to happen" and ordered the return of the mifepristone and misoprostol pills from the Customs Service. That same day, in response to a previously prepared appeal from the Bush administration, the Second Circuit Court of Appeals met in a three-judge panel, including "Judge John Walker, President Bush's first cousin; Daniel Mahoney, former chair of the strongly anti-choice New York State Conservative Party, and Frank Altimari, a Reagan appointee."[35] Not surprisingly, the court overturned the earlier finding by the district court. In response, the pro-choice coalition appealed to the U.S. Supreme Court, which in a seven to two decision on July 18, 1992 refused to return the pills and avoided ruling on the constitutional question. The next pro-choice strategy was a requirement to turn up the pressure on Hoechst-Roussel and/or to find smaller companies (anywhere) to produce the drug and somehow get the RU-486 patent transferred to a U.S. company. This tactic only became viable with the help of President Clinton.

PRESIDENT BILL CLINTON AND RU-486

Big pharma in the United States was concerned about its solvency in the early 1990s, since the drug research and approval pipeline had slowed down. Part of the blockage was attributed to Reagan era funding cuts for FDA inspection staff.[36] The lack of potential blockbusters was mainly viewed by the pharma industry as an effect of the pro-generics 1984 Hatch-Waxman legislation. Presidents Clinton and George W. Bush helped pave the way for mega-mergers affecting many of the companies covered in this book (Syntex, Searle, Pfizer, Merck, etc.). President Clinton presided over the greatest number of mergers in U.S. pharma industry, from 1994 to 1996.[37] While the Clinton administration liked to portray itself as hard-nosed on antitrust and merger issues, other analyses have suggested that with the exception of the well-publicized Microsoft case, the administration's outlook was moderate.[38]

The differences between the three Republican presidents and the Democratic one were that the Republican ones owed more to the social conservative base than did President Clinton. Thus, the arrows of favoring business and listening to social conservatives both went in the same direction, toward hurting women by failing to allow RU-486 and Plan B to proceed under the Republicans. Compared to Republicans in the White House, President Clinton was about as pro-business as they were and willing to cut deals with social conservatives if other objectives, such as welfare reform, could be achieved. Where he differed most strongly was in wanting to keep much of the feminist bloc voting for him. The following discussion shows how the Clinton administration's strategies in the struggle to make

RU-486 available in the United States ultimately benefited both women and the Hoechst-Roussel company.

An important opening in the political opportunity structure occurred when President Clinton took office with a Democratic Congress (1993–1995). On January 22, 1993 (*Roe v Wade*'s 20th anniversary) and two days after his swearing-in, President Clinton directed Health and Human Services (HHS) secretary Donna Shalala to take two important actions toward making RU-486 available in the United States. The first was to put a notice in the *Federal Register* that the administration was taking steps to rescind FDA Import Alert 66-47, the Automatic Detention of Abortifacient Drugs. Toward that end, Secretary Shalala directed the FDA "to initiate an immediate and thorough review of the health and safety implications of the potential import of RU-486 for personal use," with the findings to be reported to her.[39] If no evidence were found to support the import ban, it would be rescinded. This open process of appropriate notice in the *Federal Register* was in direct contrast to the Bush administration's procedures. In early 1993, FDA officials and HHS secretary Donna E. Shalala began negotiations with Hoechst-Roussel and the Population Council, which had also been negotiating on the issue. In April 1993, the White House announced that the French company would agree to transfer the rights to RU-486 to the Population Council so that the council could conduct clinical trials and find a U.S. manufacturer.[40] One year later, the details had not been worked out and only after Secretary Shalala set a deadline of May 15, 1994 was a formal agreement signed. The quest for a manufacturer was the crucial issue.

Advocacy and research groups started two sets of efforts to bring mifepristone to the United States by finding a manufacturer for it. One strategy involved Lawrence Lader and his organization, Abortion Rights Mobilization (ARM). He began working contacts in China, who had been illegally copying the RU-486 pill even before it was put on the French market, as early as 1983. He got the head of the RU-486 distribution program in China, a doctor at Peking Union Medical College, to send some pills to U.S. doctors so that their formulary could be compared with the French pills that Lader had acquired before the *Benten* lawsuit.[41] Lader also got the Chinese doctor to agree to provide U.S. doctors with the results of the Chinese clinical testing.[42] However, Lader noted that "FDA contacts implied that they would have less faith in a Chinese version than in a US-made copy of it."[43] Lader then sought the help of Dr. Chang of the Worcester Foundation, one of the inventors of the Pill, and received names of some potentially cooperative U.S.-based scientists. An unnamed scientist was found, to be supervised by anti-progestin expert Dr. David Horne from Columbia University. ARM, Lader's organization, covered "all bills, checks and mail by that name alone." Some financial support was also forthcoming from a "long-time pro-choice foundation based in the Midwest."[44] Lader also states that clinical disbursement of free pills to women in the ARM trial was declared legal by the group's lawyers. While it is illegal to sell unapproved drugs in the United States, it is not illegal to distribute them as part of clinical trials before approval. In the meantime, an ARM lawyer, Edward Costikyan, an old friend of HHS secretary Shalala's, asked whether ARM could approach the FDA even though Roussel was then in meetings with Shalala and the FDA. Her response was positive, and on January 1, 1993, ARM held a press conference aimed at pressuring Hoechst-Roussel, which had been dragging its feet, to action by stating that "if Roussel kept delaying, we would urge the US government to seize its patent."[45] Patent seizures are a rare process in the United States, usually invoked only in national emergencies or as wartime acquisitions. ARM also found a helpful ally in Representative Ron Wyden of Oregon, who had sponsored unsuccessful legislation to overturn the FDA import ban on RU-486. As chair of the House subcommittee on Small Business in 1993, he was willing to file a bill to strip Hoechst's patent over RU-486 if it did not make the drug available.[46]

The second, more longterm effort on RU-486 availability was through the research institute the Population Council, which had first been involved in testing the drug on 300 women at USC starting in 1983, until Roussel backed out in 1989 (shortly after the Import Alert of June 1989) and USC ran out of pills in 1990.[47] The Population Council had obtained the Investigational New Drug (IND) approval from the FDA in 1983. Lader and the ARM took the popular mobilization route, working in particular with the Feminist Majority Foundation (FMF) and its director Eleanor Smeal to promote RU-486. The ARM–FMF message was one of showing the rise in anti-clinic violence in 1993–1994 and promoting RU-486 as a way to avoid dangerous abortion clinics. Instead, women would obtain the pill in a doctor's office and then take it at home, later returning to the office for medical follow-up. Another strategy practiced by the FMF, particularly after 1989 and the U.S. Supreme Court *Webster* decision, was the Web of Influence campaign in which the FMF publicized the U.S. companies doing business with Hoechst-Roussel and asked Americans to write letters to those companies indicating their support of their products and of mifepristone's availability in the United States. Another was that the FMF sent hundreds of thousands of petitions from Americans to both the Hoechst office in New Jersey and the French Roussel Uclaf offices between 1989 and 1992.[48] In his 1995 book, Lader described the efforts of ARM to publicly pressure Hoechst as helpful and implied a strong profit motive on the part of the Population Council's interest in RU-486.[49] Ultimately, both groups were included in the meetings between the FDA and HHS secretary Donna Shalala.

On April 20, 1993, FDA head Dr. David Kessler announced that Roussel Uclaf was willing to give the Council 2000 pills and its clinical data on RU-486. As Judith Johnson reported in the Congressional Research Service (CRS) brief on RU-486, in September 1993, the Institute of Medicine released its report, *Clinical Applications of Mifepristone RU-486 and Other Antiprogestins,* funded by the Henry J. Kaiser Family Foundation. What is fascinating because it so rarely happens in the U.S. pharma system, rigged as it is against foreign competitors, is that the institute recommended that that the FDA use the French data for considering the drug application, "to determine whether the French trials met US regulatory requirements."[50] Not surprisingly, given the activities of social conservatives in the second policy punctuation on reproductive drugs, they immediately responded to this recommendation. The recommendation was to urge the FDA not to rely on foreign data.[51] This response pushed the FDA to conduct U.S.-based trials of mifepristone so that American data could be added to the foreign studies.

The Population Council announced that it was willing to share its IND for mifepristone with ARM so that the latter would not have to spend time and effort getting that achieved. However, the Council also intended to pursue its own source of the drug in the United States (after the Roussel pills in the trial ran out). Lader and the ARM worked to get FDA approval in May 1993 for ARM to develop a clinical trial protocol to be based in Virginia. On April 20, 1994, ARM signed a contract with a British lab to produce more pills from the version that Dr. Horne and the other ARM scientists had already produced.[52]

On April 14, 1994, HHS secretary Donna Shalala and FDA commissioner Kessler met with Hoechst-Roussel and gave them a deadline of May 15, 1994 by which to agree to allow the Population Council to go ahead with FDA approval for mifepristone or that presumably the Clinton administration would force the issue. On May 16, 1994, Secretary Shalala announced that Hoechst-Roussel had agreed to turn over its RU-486 patent to the Population Council without charge and all the clinical data it possessed as well. The Population Council decided not to work with ARM and proceeded on its own.[53] It still had only limited supplies of RU-486 provided by Roussel and needed to find another manufacturer. From October 1994 to September 1995, the Population Council conducted studies on 2121 women in the United States, funded by George Soros's Open Society Institute and the Kaiser Family Foundation.[54] Roussel was providing pills for the Population Council tests.

On March 18, 1996, the Population Council filed a new drug application for mifepristone (to be combined with misoprostol), using the data from the nearly 2500 French women provided by Roussel and its own data on more than 2100 women.[55] On July 19, 1996, the Advisory Committee on Reproductive

Health of the FDA's Center for Drug Evaluation and Research recommended that the FDA approve mifepristone in combination with misoprostol as an effective way to end pregnancies of up to seven weeks gestation.[56] As Johnson notes, the FDA took the unusual step of not releasing the committee members' names for fear of retribution. The committee's recommendation also required close medical supervision of the provision of mifepristone, and thus that it should only be provided directly by doctors in their offices. On September 18, 1996, the FDA issued an approvable letter to the Population Council for RU-486 with misoprostol (still unavailable, due to its patent status with Searle). The approvable letter is a signal sent by the FDA to the company (or to the Population Council in this unusual case) that it wants more information on a particular aspect of the process.[57] In this case, the FDA wanted more information about the manufacturer and labeling for mifepristone. Here, the FDA was in the exact same position as the Population Council. While ARM had initially requested FDA approval to begin testing in 1993, this permission was not granted until 1996. ARM said it had produced up to 10,000 pills, likely through British and Chinese sources, to use in tests. It had produced an original pill in an underground lab just outside of Westchester, New York.[58] The ARM tests were funded by the John Merck Foundation.[59]

The Population Council thought it had the problem of getting a well-known manufacturer for mifepristone solved when Gedeon Richter of Hungary agreed to produce the pill for the council in 1995. The Population Council began a complicated series of steps to establish arm's-length subsidiaries that could handle marketing and hopefully manufacturing mifepristone, if a U.S. source could be found. The first subsidiary was named Advances in Health Technology (AHT). It soon ran into trouble because the man chosen on a council board member's recommendation to head AHT, Joseph Pike, was a disbarred North Carolina lawyer who had not divulged his status. Since he was supposed to head the efforts by the council's subsidiary to obtain a U.S. manufacturer and the bulk of funding, his loss to the project had a large effect. This impact was especially true because by 1997 Pike had raised 27 million dollars in funding for the project, including 6 million dollars of his own.[60] While the Population Council sued Pike, the two sides settled when Pike sold his interest in AHT to its next iteration, Advances for Choice.[61] Over the next two years, the subsidiary name changed to Neogen and then ultimately the Population Council announced in 1999 that it would work with the Danco company, incorporated in the Caymans. Danco is still listed as the company providing mifepristone in the United States.[62]

In the meantime, the mifepristone advocacy community had established a link with Hua Lian Pharmaceuticals, outside Shanghai. The Concept Foundation, an arm's-length foundation funded by Rockefeller and others and headquartered in Bangkok, also provided some funding at this stage. In 1998, it was reported that, "RU-486 has been a key ingredient in China's population control strategy for years. Of the estimated 10 million abortions performed annually in China, about half are carried out with RU-486, said Gao Ersheng, director of the Shanghai Institute of Planned Parenthood Research. . . . Hua Lian has been making RU-486 for at least nine years, one of three companies in China that manufacture the drug."[63] Also interesting is the fact that the World Health Organization (WHO) was carrying out trials in the 1980s with a drug that had not yet been approved by the FDA.

In 1997, in short order a few events happened, all linked to each other and the ultimate fate of RU-486. In April 1997, Hoechst (which had bought all of Roussel) announced it would cease production of RU-486, justified in part by a large anti-choice boycott of the company's Allegra drug.[64] It transferred its French patent rights and remaining stock to Dr. Edouard Sakiz, one of the scientists who invented RU-486 and former head of Roussel. His new company, Exelgyn, is still the European manufacturer of mifepristone. In February 1997, Gedeon Richter backed out of its contract with the Population Council to produce mifepristone. It is likely that by that date the company knew about the impending Hoechst deal and decided to remove itself from the scenario. The Population Council was furious and tried unsuccessfully to sue the Hungarian company to force it to comply with the contract. In the meantime, another deal moved things forward in the United States with Hoechst.

Presumably also sweetening the pot for Hoechst was the fact that it bought Marion Merrell Dow in 1995, under the eyes of the Clinton administration. Lawrence Lader wrote that the event turning the Hoechst company's years of intransigence around when they finally agreed to donate the patent rights in 1994 was that "I suspect that President Clinton used some sort of economic prod."[65] Marion Merrell Dow was formed when the Dow Chemical Company bought Richardson-Merrell in 1980. Richardson-Merrell was previously discussed for its desire to push thalidomide onto the U.S. market in the 1960s, and to bully Dr. Frances Kelsey out of the FDA. Richardson-Merrell-Dow then bought Marion Laboratories in 1989. At the time, "Marion Laboratories was outperforming all other US drug stocks by a factor of 2.5," and "had the highest sales and profit per employee of any company traded on the New York Stock Exchange." This offer "made 300 of Marion's employees millionaires." It also made Marion Merrell Dow the fifth largest drug company in the United States based on sales.[66] Thus, Hoechst did quite well in the deal, getting rid of a patent it did not want and acquiring a profitable U.S.-based company.

Again in February 2000, the FDA issued another approvable letter for mifepristone, but no further action was taken. Many speculated that as in 1996 when those in the medical community admitted that RU-486 was being held up in anticipation of the 1996 presidential elections, the same was true in 2000. As is also known, Searle's patent for Cytotec (misoprostol) expired in July 2000. Jane Henney, M.D., was President Clinton's nominee to head the FDA after Dr. David Kessler resigned in 1998. She was grilled by conservative senators, including Don Nickles (OK) who required the promise that she "would not solicit a US-based manufacturer for RU-486."[67] However, she announced its approval for prescription status for those 18 and older on September 28, 2000.[68] In November 2000, the first shipments of RU-486 made in China under the patent to the Population Council arrived in the United States and were sent to physicians.

The Danco–Population Council link is still the partnership of record for distributing mifepristone in the United States and Exelgyn is the European distributor. Another event has taken place whereby the mifepristone–misoprostol combination is available through global connections, including the Population Council, Planned Parenthood, and the WHO. In 2003, Dr. Beverly Winikoff, M.D., formed Gynuity Health Projects, an organization devoted to helping get women's reproductive drugs more available on the global market. Dr. Winikoff had previously been director of Reproductive Health at the Population Council for 25 years.[69] Among Gynuity's key projects is getting the RU-486/misoprostol regimen widely available and it has been successful in this around the globe, although at present time only about 50 countries have approved it. Due to Gynuity's and the Population Council's connections, the WHO approved RU-486 with misoprostol for its global formulary in 2004.

CONCLUSION

The politics surrounding the development of a mifepristone/misoprostol regime for the United States involved quirks surrounding the history of both drugs. While misoprostol (licensed to Searle as Cytotec until 2000) had been available in the United States since the 1970s, mifepristone was discovered in France in the early 1980s. Similarly, while companies decried the notion that either mifepristone or misoprostol could be important (profitable) enough to warrant supposedly putting their other drugs at risk for an anti-choice boycott, those that have ultimately chosen to market reproductive drugs have benefitted handsomely. Consistent with the discussion of the Pill, it was shown that politicians and pharma companies interchangeably used financial interest or social conservative threats to cover their own lack of enthusiasm for helping women. Perhaps most surprisingly, Searle, which had first gotten FDA approval of the Pill and made billions from it, was not willing to be helpful in the mifepristone fight by making misoprostol available as part of the formulary.

The discussion in this chapter has shown the relevance of the theories of the iron triangle, punctuated equilibrium (as demonstrated by the window of opportunity during the Clinton administrations), and access to the state and allies (for both pro-choice and antichoice groups) as per Tarrow's formulation. The efforts to bring in RU-486 and then to find manufacturers and/or distributors all took place during the second punctuation of women's reproductive policies. These efforts are thus framed in a period of overall unfriendliness to women's access to reproductive drugs, and the RU-486 struggle is evidence of it. The struggles began in the 1989 with the FDA adding RU-486 to the Import Alert list when conservative members of Congress exerted pressure. At the time, Frank Young, a Reagan appointee, was FDA Commissioner. The tactics of the FDA on this event were a layering into the federal government, the same tactics that were used during the Comstock era to prevent contraceptive imports. The struggles to get RU-486 in the United States continued in the 1990s when no U.S. firm could be found to manufacture it, and Hoechst-Roussel refused to sell it in the United States, buckling to social conservative pressure. The prevailing discourse of the George H. W. Bush administration was based on his own conversion to pro-life policies while he was Ronald Reagan's vice president.

Upon the inauguration of President Clinton in 1993, the public discourse around women's reproductive rights immediately changed. Among his first acts was the rescission of the Reagan and Bush anti-abortion executive orders, and giving HHS secretary Donna Shalala the brief to restart negotiations with Hoechst-Roussel. The administration was helpful in this regard and in ultimately getting the mifepristone patent turned over to the Population Council. Work by the Population Council, Lawrence Lader, and Eleanor Smeal was required to find a Chinese manufacturer for the pill. Another example of the layering of strategies is shown when Lader adopted Margaret Sanger's 1936 tactic of alerting Customs officials to the import of banned material and generating court actions from this. Unfortunately, Lader's court challenge took place in 1992, with the appellate and Supreme courts under the thumb of Ronald Reagan and George H. W. Bush.

The roles of Lawrence Lader, Eleanor Smeal, and then the CRLP were to try to effect a discursive shift about the reproductive rights of women, most prominently under the administration of George H. W. Bush. The push for RU-486 was that Reagan- and Bush-era court appointees and their tolerance of anti-choice activism made reproductive clinics an unsafe place for women to go for surgical abortions. The National Organization for Women, the FMF's parent organization, had been engaged in a lawsuit against Joseph Scheidler, head of the Pro-Life Action League, since 1987. The CRLP took the *Benten* case to contribute to a discursive moment during the unfriendly Bush administration when the public platform could be used to show the unfairness of Bush's policies toward women.

The Clinton administration's FDA was mostly friendly toward women's rights, with the exception being the abstinence-based policies attached to welfare reform. Both RU-486 and Preven, the combination formula for emergency contraception, were approved under Clinton-appointed FDA commissioners, first David Kessler until 1998 and then Jane Henney. Unfortunately, Plan B did not get submitted to the FDA in time to be approved by Jane Henney. It then went through twists and turns under the George W. Bush administration's FDA, a thoroughly different creature with three different commissioners.

NOTES

1. "Misoprostol Alone," *Medical Abortion*, http://www.medicationabortion.com/misoprostol/index.html.

2. Ibid.

3. Loren Stein, "Un-Informed Consent," *Metro Active*, http://www.sciencebasedbirth.com/safety_issues01/CytotecDeathOakland.htm.

4. Judith A. Johnson, "Abortion: Termination of Early Pregnancy with RU-486 (Mifepristone)," *CRS Report for Congress*, Order Code RL 30866 (Washington, DC: Congressional Research Service, February 23, 2001), 9, 11, http://www.law.umaryland.edu/marshall/crsreports/crsdocuments/RL30866.pdf.

5. Stein, "Un-Informed Consent."

6. Johnson, "Abortion," 21–22.

7. "G. D. Searle & Co. History: Company History," *Funding Universe*, http://www.fundinguniverse.com/company-histories/g-d-searle-co-history/.

8. Amanda Melpolder, *The Bitterest Pill: How Drug Companies Fail to Protect Women and How Lawsuits Save Their Lives* (New York: Center for Justice and Democracy, 2008), 12, http://centerjd.org/content/study-bitterest-pill-%E2%80%93-how-drug-companies-fail-protect-women-and-how-lawsuits-save-their.

9. "Monsanto's Dark History, 1901–2011," *BestMeal.info*, http://bestmeal.info/monsanto/company-history.shtml/.

10. Julie Hogan, "The Life of the Abortion Pill in the US," *LEDA at Harvard Law School*, fts. 127, 185–88, http://leda.law.harvard.edu/leda/data/247/Hogan,_Julie.pdf.

11. Letter from Sandra Arnold, vice president of the Population Council, October 25, 1999, in FDA files concerning RU-486, www.fda.gov/cder/archives/mifepristone.

12. "Resolution Calling for the Reform of the FDA" *ALEC Exposed*, http://alecexposed.org/w/images/d/d7/5E0-Resolution_Calling_for_the_Reform_of_the_Food_and_Drug_Administration_Exposed.pdf.

13. "History," *American Legislative Exchange Council (ALEC)*, http://www.alec.org/about-alec/history/.

14. Wendell Potter, "ALEC Exposed: Sabotaging Healthcare," *The Nation*, July 12, 2011, http://wendellpotter.com/2011/07/alec-exposed-sabotaging-healthcare/.

15. Ibid.

16. "History," *ALEC*.

17. Ibid.

18. Fred Clarkson, "Takin' It to the States: The Rise of Conservative State Level Think Tanks," *The Public Eye* XIII, nos. 2–3 (Summer/Fall 1999), http://www.publiceye.org/magazine/v13n2-3/PE_V13_N2-3.pdf.

19. "Monsanto's Dark History," *BestMeal.info*.

20. Kathi E. Hanna, *Biomedical Politics* (Washington, DC: Institute of Medicine, National Academy Press, 1991), 69.

21. Hogan, "The Life of the Abortion Pill," Part III.

22. Ibid., ft. 538.

23. "Monsanto's Dark History," *BestMeal.info*.

24. Margaret Talbot, "The Little White Bombshell: Why RU-486 Could Change Everything About Abortion," *The New York Times Magazine*, July 11, 1999, 5–7, http://www.newamerica.net/node/5733.

25. Denise Chicoine, "RU-486 in the United States and Great Britain: A Case Study in Gender Bias," *Boston College International and Comparative Law Review* 16, no. 1 (1993): 81–113, http://lawdigitalcommons.bc.edu/iclr/vol16/iss1/4/.

26. Hogan, "The Life of the Abortion Pill," Part IV.

27. Ibid.

28. Chicoine, "RU-486 in the United States," 95.

29. Lynda Crouse, "*Benten v. Kessler:* The Time for Uniformity in the Application of Section 553 of the Administrative Procedure Act has Come," *The American University Administrative Law Journal* 7 (Summer 1993): 344–71.

30. Daniel Carpenter, *Reputation and Power: Organizational Image and Pharmaceutical Regulation at the FDA* (Princeton, NJ: Princeton University Press, 2010), 440.

31. Chicoine, "RU-486 in the United States," 94–98.

32. Ibid.

33. Lawrence Lader, *A Private Matter: RU-486 and the Abortion Crisis* (Amherst, NY: Prometheus Books, 1995), 133–36.

34. Ibid., 137.

35. Ibid., 137–38.

36. Stephen Ceccoli, *Pill Politics: Drugs and the FDA* (Boulder, CO: Lynne Rienner, 2003), 104.

37. David J. Ravenscraft and William F. Long, "Paths to Creating Value in Pharmaceutical Mergers," in *Mergers and Productivity*, ed. Steven N. Kaplan (Chicago, IL: University of Chicago Press, 2000), 287–326.

38. Thomas B. Leary, "The Essential Stability of Merger Policy in the United States," *Guidelines for Merger Remedies: Prospects and Principles* (Paris: U.S. Federal Trade Commission, January 17, 2002), http://www.ftc.gov/speeches/leary/learyuseu.shtm and Sara Fisher Ellison and Wallace P. Mullin, "Gradual Incorporation of Information: Pharmaceutical Stocks and the Evolution of President Clinton's Health Care Reform," *Journal of Law and Economics* XLIV, no. 1 (April 2001): 89–129, http://time.dufe.edu.cn/jingjiwencong/waiwenziliao1/004102.web.pdf.

39. Johnson, "Abortion," 2–3.

40. Karen Young Kreeger, "Some Researchers Are Pleased, Others Indifferent, RU-486 Moves toward Ready Availability in the US," *The Scientist* 8, no.16 (August 22, 1994): 1.

41. *Benten v. Kessler,* 799 F. Supp. 281, 1992 (U.S. District Court).

42. Lader, *A Private Matter,* 141–42.

43. Ibid., 143.

44. Ibid., 142–46.

45. Ibid., 147–49.

46. Ibid., 149.

47. Johnson, "Abortion," 2–3.

48. Hogan, "The Life of the Abortion Pill," ft. 291.

49. Lader, *A Private Matter.*

50. Johnson, "Abortion," 5.

51. Ibid.

52. Lader, *A Private Matter,* 151–62.

53. Ibid., 160–61.

54. Johnson, "Abortion," 5.

55. Ibid., 5.

56. Ibid., 6.

57. Ibid., 5.

58. Talbot, "The Little White Bombshell," 5–7.

59. Hogan, "The Life of the Abortion Pill," ft. 564 and Johnson, "Abortion," ft. 21.

60. Johnson, "Abortion." ft. 32.

61. Ibid.

62. Ibid., 7.

63. Philip P. Pan, "Chinese to Make RU-486 for US," *Washington Post,* October 12, 2000, A1, www.washingtonpost.com.

64. Johnson, "Abortion." 7.

65. Lader, *A Private Matter,* 157.

66. Dick Davis, "Marion Laboratories Predicted to Outperform All Drug Stocks," *St. Petersburg Times,* June 18, 2009 and "Hoechst Agrees to Buy Marion Merrell Dow/Acquisition worth $7 Billion," www.sftimes.com.

67. Jean Reith Schroedel and Tanya Buhler Corbin, "Gender Relations and Institutional Conflict over Mifepristone," *Women & Politics* 24, no. 3 (2002): 49.

68. Hogan, "The Life of the Abortion Pill," 32.

69. "About Us: Beverly Winikoff," *Gynuity Health Projects,* http://gynuity.org/about/staff/winikoff/.

6

The "Morning-After Pill," Plan B (Levonorgestrel) Formulation

The crux of this chapter concerns changes from Food and Drug Administration (FDA) practices under President Clinton to those under President Bush, specifically regarding over-the-counter (OTC) status for Plan B. The Clinton administration had approved the combination emergency contraceptive pill (EC) called Preven, the progestin-only Plan B and RU-486, on prescription-only bases from 1998 to 2000. Conversely, the Bush administration took from 2003 to 2006 to approve Plan B OTC for 18 year olds and over. Led by Commissioner Jane Henney, the FDA approved Plan B as a prescription-based drug in 1999 and suggested to the company (then Barr Laboratories) that it might be able to submit an application to move it to OTC status.

Part of the problem in the Bush administration was that there was no FDA commissioner from 2001 until 2002, when Dr. Mark McClellan was confirmed. McClellan held the post from 2002 to 2004, then Dr. Lester B. Crawford (a veterinarian) from 2004 to 2005, and then Dr. Andrew von Eschenbach from 2005 to 2009. Both McClellan and von Eschenbach had deep Texas roots, McClellan as part of a Texas political family and von Eschenbach having spent much of his career as a urologist at the MD Anderson Cancer Center at the University of Texas (beginning in 1976). He was with the cancer center until President George W. Bush appointed him as director of the National Cancer Institute (in the Department of Health and Human Services) in 2001. Both Crawford, who had previously been in four positions at the FDA, and von Eschenbach were criticized as FDA commissioners for being overly risk-averse.[1] Senator Barbara Mikulski characterized Crawford's one-year chairmanship as "tepid and weak."[2] It is clear that neither Lester Crawford nor von Eschenbach were strong advocates for switching Plan B to OTC status.

The relevant theoretical foundations for this chapter are historical institutionalism, discursive institutionalism, feminist interpretations of them, Tarrow's political opportunity structure, and the models of Baumgartner and Jones's punctuated equilibrium and Burnham's political realignments. In terms of historical institutionalism, Hacker's characterization of increased social risk tolerated by the U.S. health-delivery system since the 1980s is relevant to this discussion of increased risk to U.S. women since the beginning of the Republican realignment on reproductive rights issues. Streeck and Thelen's use of the term "conversion" is also relevant, as is the layering concept of later reforms onto earlier ones. An example of layering was the Gore–Clinton's "reinventing-government" initiative to expedite the workings of bureaucracy and how it was placed on top of changes already occurring at the FDA.[3]

Regarding the workings of the FDA in the 1990s as opposed to 2000–2008, the former term saw many drugs approved, quickly. In addition to the three reproductive drugs approved from 1998 to 2000, Vioxx, which is also relevant to this study, was approved in May 1999. Vioxx's approval was rescinded due to side effects in 2005, and Gardasil became Merck's blockbuster of choice.

In 1992, the Prescription Drug User Fee Act (PDUFA) was passed while Dr. David Kessler was FDA commissioner. Kessler was the first commissioner to require Senate confirmation, served both Presidents George H. W. Bush and Clinton, and was a cheerleader for expanding the FDA's authority and efficiency in decision-making. In 1997, FDA deputy commissioner Michael Friedman testified to the U.S. House Commerce Committee to support the upcoming renewal of PDUFA. His remarks centered on the progress that the FDA had been able to make under the user-fee regime assessed to pharma companies, whereby the FDA increased its staff. Deputy Commissioner Friedman stated that because of increased staff, the FDA had improved its approval time to six months or less on breakthrough (new molecular entity [NME]) drugs and one year or less on all other drugs. He also stated that, "the number of NMEs approved each year is regarded as a real indication of meaningful medical progress. Last year, that progress was exceptional: FDA approved 53 NMEs, the most ever and nearly twice as many as any year before."[4]

Unlike Daniel Carpenter, who favors more gradualist historical institutionalist explanations, Stephen Ceccoli has applied the punctuated equilibrium model to the FDA. The punctuated equilibrium model is appropriate for explaining the severe shifts in receptivity to women's reproductive drugs across Democratic and Republican administrations, particularly after 1980. During the George W. Bush presidency, OTC status for Plan B was delayed until midway in his second term. On the other hand, Gardasil sailed through FDA approval in a few months, so as to fill Merck's coffers. While Plan B was safe and effective, serious concerns about Gardasil remain. Regarding Tarrow's framework, women had powerful allies within the administration, therefore access to the state, in the form of Health and Human Services secretary Donna Shalala under President Clinton. Under President George W. Bush, they did not. Ultimately, pro-Plan B advocacy groups were able to call on senators, including Hillary Clinton, Patty Murray, Dianne Feinstein, Barbara Boxer, and Barbara Mikulski, to put holds on the nominations of Lester Crawford and then Andrew von Eschenbach as FDA commissioners. Another extremely important alliance between pro-choice groups was the work done by the Center for Reproductive Rights to sue the FDA for a decision on OTC Plan B access in 2006. Finally, discursive institutionalism as theorized by Lombardo, Meier, and Verloo is important to this analysis, regarding the central question of whether gender equality is a fundamental concept in various policy fields. With regard to getting Plan B OTC only for 18 year olds and over (lowered by one year in 2009), Lombardo et al.'s characterization of the policy dialogue and impact as fixing, is fitting in which the right is understood to be frozen at a particular point and will not be expanded. Health and Human Services Secretary Kathleen Sebelius's refusal to reopen the question of OTC for all in December 2011 confirms the notion of fixing the concept of equality through Plan B as OTC only for women 17 and older.[5]

DEVELOPMENT OF EMERGENCY CONTRACEPTION

As with the contraceptive pill and scientific knowledge about the use of hormones to prevent pregnancy in the 1920s, similar tests were performed by veterinarians at the time to prevent pregnancy after animal coitus.[6] Charlotte Ellertson states that although there were scattered reports of high-dosage hormones being used for after-the-fact contraception in the 1940s, the first published study emerged from the Netherlands in the 1960s.[7] High-dosage combinations of estrogen pills were used in non-U.S. studies, including DES (estrogen diethylstilbestrol). In the 1970s, DES was linked to vaginal cancer in the daughters of women who had taken the drug.[8] That outcome plus side effects from the estrogen-only pills led to studies with a combination of synthetic estrogen plus progestin. The studies using high dosages of synthetic estrogen and progestin used a pill that was on the market at the time, Ovral. The experimental dosage for EC included two doses of pills containing a combination of estrogen and progestin, with each dose containing 100 micrograms of ethinyl estradiol and 1.0 milligrams of norgestrel.[9] Four pills in total were taken, 2 within 72 hours after unprotected sex and the other 2 within 12 hours; the total dosage then was 200 micrograms of estradiol and 2.0 milligrams of norgestrel (equivalent to 1.0 milligrams of levonorgestrel, the Plan B drug). Both norgestrel and levonorgestrel are second-generation progestins, in which the enhancement effects of taking male-based hormones are minimized as much as possible.

Canadian reproductive endocrinologist Dr. Albert Yuzpe conducted studies using the high-dosage Ovral pills from 1970 to 1972 and reported success. One of the key factors emphasized was the progestin norgestrel, which prevented implantation of the fertilized egg.[10] The Yuzpe method, as it came to be known, showed 75 percent effectiveness.[11] Very soon, the Yuzpe method gained favor, because the addition of progestin (norgestrel) to the regimen lessened side effects and increased effectiveness from the estrogen-only methods. Ellertson notes that in the 1970s, studies were done in Latin America using different levels of levonorgestrel, varying from 150 to 400 micrograms (0.0015 to 0.4 milligrams) per tablet. This regimen was being tested more as an ongoing postcoital formulation for women who had intercourse four times per month or fewer.[12] While these studies took place in Latin America in the 1970s, Ellertson has noted that the first large study of levonorgestrel took place in Hong Kong in the early 1990s, and a WHO (World Health Organization) trial began in 1991.[13] These studies used the standard dosage adopted in Plan B, the two 0.75 milligrams dosage pills, taken 12 hours apart. The WHO study showed the superior effectiveness of the progestin-only formulation, and that the Yuzpe combination of four Ovral pills was only about as effective as a dose of mifepristone.[14] As was previously discussed, mifepristone is not considered sufficiently effective when taken alone.

From the examples of the combination and progestin-only EC formulations, we see that FDA requirement that U.S. data be used for approvals is not always met. In the previous discussion of RU-486, it was shown that Hoechst-Roussel turned over its French data to the FDA to help expedite approval. With respect to EC, clinical testing occurred mostly outside the United States. Similarly, drugs can be put on the WHO's essential medicines list, created in 1977 and updated every two years.[15] This list contains about 350 drugs. In 1979, the Yuzpe method for EC was added to the essential medicines list, 18 years before FDA approval. The specific combination of Ovral pills was added to the WHO list with the understanding that the dosage was for EC, and was publicly identified as off-label usage. Levonorgestrel in the formulation of two pills at 0.75 milligrams each was added to the WHO's essential medicines list in 1999.[16] In 2002, the levonorgestrel-only formulation superseded the Ovral/Yuzpe combination formula on the WHO's list.

In 1997, the FDA approved the Yuzpe method as an off-label use of the specific combination of Ovral birth-control pills. One year later, the dedicated product Preven for EC use only was approved by the FDA. The Preven kit contained four high-dosage birth-control pills, an information packet, and a home pregnancy test.[17] In 1995, a women's health corporation, Gynetics, was formed to "develop and market pharmaceutical products and medical devices to advance the health-care of women, which included the marketing of Preven."[18] A description of the Barr Company states that Gynetics was the marketing organization and Barr the manufacturer for Preven.[19] The International Consortium for Emergency Contraception was formed in 1996, and lists 30 pro-choice organizations as partners on its website.[20] In 2004, Barr Laboratories discontinued the manufacturing of Preven.

Plan B, the dedicated two levonorgestrel-pill formula for EC, was approved for prescription-only use in 1999 by the FDA. At the time, it was suggested to the Women's Capital Corporation that it could resubmit an application for OTC use. The New Drug Application was filed by Barr Laboratories in 2003 to allow Plan B to be approved for OTC use. It had also developed a generic version of Plan B in 2003.

More specifics about the way in which OTC status for Plan B was treated as a political football across various FDA heads in the George W. Bush administrations are as follows. It has been noted that "a resounding majority of scientific reviewers voted in favor of OTC status for (Plan B) EC in the winter of 2003. But Steven Galson, acting director of the FDA's Center for Drug Evaluation and Research, rejected their advice in May 2004, calling OTC status 'not approvable.'"[21] His official statement that girls under 16 should not have OTC access was based on the notion that women under 16 should consult with a doctor.[22] Galson was clearly rewarded for his stance by being promoted from deputy director of the Committee for Drug Evaluation and Research at FDA to being its director in 2005 and then acting Surgeon General from 2007 to 2009. By that time, as of 2004, Barr Laboratories had bought out the Women's Capital Corporation and was encouraged to submit a revised proposal, which it did in July 2004, proposing prescription-only access for women under 16 and OTC status for those over 16. The decision-making deadline of January 2005 came and went.

In August 2005, FDA Commissioner Lester Crawford "agreed that science supported OTC access for women over 17," but asked for more time to consider the request for prescription status for women under 16. This event precipitated the departure of Dr. Susan Wood, Director of the FDA Office of Women's Health. While Lester Crawford's Senate confirmation had been held up until August 2005 in an effort led by Senators Hillary Clinton and Patty Murray, they allowed it to go through on his assurance that OTC status was imminent. Given that one year later, no such decision had been made, it was clear that the senators had not been told the truth. Lester Crawford resigned two months after Dr. Wood, in October 2005, as did Frank Davidoff, who had been on the FDA's Nonprescription Drugs Advisory Committee. Davidoff's resignation statement concluded his wish to leave an organization "that is capable of making such an important decision so flagrantly on the basis of political influence."[23] Another example of undue influence was shown by one FDA advisor, Dr. David Hager, writing a minority report against FDA approval of Plan B. He did so in response to being asked by an unnamed person. Hager is a gynecologist notorious for incorporating literal biblical understandings into his practice.[24]

In November 2005, the Government Accountability Office (GAO) report blew the protective cover off the Bush administration's track record on interference with the FDA over the EC decision (regarding both potential OTC provision and prescriptions for minors). It stated that "high-level FDA management was more involved than usual in the review process, and that the non-approval decision, according to some within the FDA, had been made months before the FDA staff had completed their review."[25] Even more egregious was the fact that the political influence was specifically aimed at Plan B OTC status. The GAO report noted that there were 67 drugs considered by the FDA for a status change from prescription to OTC from 1994 to 2004. Plan B was the only drug to be denied the new status after a positive committee evaluation.[26]

In 2005, the Center for Reproductive Rights (CRR, having changed its name in 2003 from the Center for Reproductive Law and Policy) filed suit against the Bush administration. The lawsuit was specifically based on the FDA having passed its own time frame for a decision on the matter, after FDA Commissioner Lester Crawford had been confirmed in summer 2005 on the basis of promising the expedited review for OTC status that had been left hanging since 2003.[27] In essence, a tag-team approach was used whereby CRR brought suit against the FDA and Senators Hillary Clinton, Patty Murray, Dianne Feinstein, and Barbara Boxer worked to publicize the FDA's obstruction of its own processes. One important piece of evidence uncovered in the CRR lawsuit was that

> A recent deposition of a senior FDA official by the Center for Reproductive Rights indicates the White House was exerting influence on the FDA regarding Plan B in order to "appease the administration's constituents." That admission was one of the bases of our decision to request the White House subpoena, however, the government has now asked that the subpoena hearing be postponed.[28]

After FDA Commissioner Crawford's resignation, Dr. Andrew von Eschenbach, head of the National Cancer Institute since 2001, was tapped for the FDA's acting commissioner position and slated for Senate confirmation. Senators Clinton and Murray had vowed not to back down again as they had with regard to Crawford in summer 2005. Based on the pressure successfully exerted by CRR and the two senators, the Bush administration backed down, agreeing to change Plan B to OTC status for women 18 years of age and older. An article in *Time* noted that "the FDA considered exactly the same studies when it approved the drug (in 2006) as it did when it denied the drug over-the-counter sales in 2003."[29] In other words, once the president decided to move forward, lack of data concerning younger women was not a problem.

In early 2009, CRR filed another lawsuit against the FDA in district court in New York. The lawsuit stated that neither scientific procedure nor the FDA's promises to review OTC status for women 16 and over supported the continued regime of OTC status only for those 18 and over. District court judge Korman agreed, rebuking the FDA for not following its own procedures. The judge noted the "unusual involvement of the White House in the Plan B decision-making process."[30] Judge Korman ruled that Barr Laboratories could pursue approval for OTC status for young women 17 and older, remanding the decision back to the FDA. The FDA accomplished the status change on April 22, 2009, to allow those 17 and older in the OTC regime.

EC ACCESS AS A STATE-BASED STRUGGLE

Doan and Williams have stated that the bulk of morality policymaking belongs to the states.[31] This is also true for criminal law in the United States. The combination means that policy legislatively defined as morality can be contested and criminalized at the state level. The struggle for access to OTC EC has been played out largely at the state level. The reasons for this setting are complex, involving legislative and regulatory competences, the division of health insurance into state-based risk pools, and the nature of the advocacy coalitions on both sides of the EC question. On the anti-choice side, groups mobilized just after the 1973 *Roe v. Wade* decision to work at returning most decision-making back to the states, thereby effectively denying a national framework of consistent reproductive rights provision. With regard to EC, groups such as Pharmacists for Life and Nurses and Physicians for Life have been crucial actors in denying services to women.

The ways to accomplish EC accessibility involved finding out which states had liberal protocols for physician–pharmacist agreements. The Program for Appropriate Technology in Health (PATH), a global health nongovernmental organization, started a pharmacy access program in 1997. It concentrated first on Washington state, which has the most liberalized state framework for collaborative practice between physicians and pharmacists. The existing protocol for collaborative practice had been in place in Washington since the 1970s. There were many upsides to the framework in PATH's eyes. The first was that it was a way to avoid the prescription-only status for EC then in place federally and in Washington. The existing framework could be adapted to specifically include EC with no regulatory or legislative changes needed. Finally, the collaborative agreement covered both "the named pharmacist and all other pharmacists who work with the client."[32] As of 1997, Washington State's collaborative practice agreement already included more than 550 pharmacists, "covering a wide range of conditions and diseases."[33]

As of 2008, it was noted that 45 states have collaborative practice agreements of some sort in place.[34] These agreements in essence allow a pharmacist to download an Internet-based form filled out by a provider, which can be a physician, physician assistant, nurse, or nurse practitioner, depending on the particular state law. Again, depending on the state, various medical issues are covered, often cancer or diabetes. The central idea behind the collaborative practice agreement is that, specific to its formulation, it can enable a client to bypass a prescription-based requirement and to bypass an age-related requirement as is so often the case for contraceptive-related provision. As noted by the National Conference of State Legislatures in July 2011, "nine states allow pharmacists to initiate emergency contraception drug therapy if they are working in collaboration with a physician, and/or after they have completed a training program in emergency contraception."[35] As of 2012, while 45 states have some sort of collaborative practice agreement in place, only nine of those states include EC in that agreement. Clearly, there is more room for pro-choice action to take place to bypass the national and state prescription age for EC.

PATH notes that the access to EC began in the densely-populated western cities of the state, and involved training providers in the use of four Ovral pills, the only method then available. In 1999, PATH developed a toolkit that included a portfolio of materials.[36] PATH then broadened its focus to the more rural eastern areas of Washington. As of 2012, PATH notes that nine states have adapted their collaborative practice agreements to include EC provision without a prescription.[37] This means that in these nine states, the federal age limit for EC without a prescription is bypassed. As of 2009, the partnership states that around 2000 women every month access Plan B through the collaborative practice agreement (going directly to pharmacies), and that while 90 pharmacies first participated in the agreement in 1997, that number was up to 300 by August 2003, with about 1900 pharmacists trained to provide the direct provision services.[38] The estimation by one pharmacist, a trainer who has worked in most of the early-adapter states, Don Downing, is that in one year alone, 1999–2000, "Washington's pharmacy program contributed to state savings of nearly $22 million in Medicaid dollars."[39]

The second state to join the collaborative framework was California through legislation passed on January 1, 2002. By that point, 70 pharmacies were already participating in the pilot project, and it coordinated most of the activities to increase public, medical, legislative, and pharmacy knowledge of how the project worked and the benefits to its expansion. Publicly-funded support for Plan B is available in California, in the amount of six packages (doses) of Plan B in one year. As of 2012, more than 900 pharmacies in the state participate in the collaborative practice framework on EC, an important figure for the nation's most populous state. In related fashion, 52 of California's 58 counties contain EC-providing pharmacies, which include 60 percent of the state's rural counties. The provision network is divided in half between independent and large chain pharmacies. Most chain store pharmacies are said to participate in the framework.[40] In addition, informal networks exist in the non-providing counties to send women to locations where Plan B can be accessed OTC.

Alaska became the second state of 2002 to include EC in its collaborative practice agreement. This state's accession into general collaborative practice happened in 2001 when general regulations were adopted by the state pharmacy board, broadened to include EC in April 2002. What is interesting about Alaska's protocol is that it allows not just physicians but also advance practice nurses to prescribe EC for pharmacists to provide.[41] As in California, the medical community and pro-EC coalition (Alaska Emergency Contraception Project, AECP) emphasized the Center for Disease Control's data of the late 1990s, which indicated that 42 percent of pregnancies in Alaska were unintended. As in Washington state, the public health argument for reducing pregnancy was a helpful frame for the pro-EC coalition to use. Many of the early-adapter states of the collaborative practice agreement on EC used a trainer, pharmacist Don Downing of Washington state to educate pharmacists. Another smart strategy was that in 2003 the project forged an alliance with the president of the Alaska Pharmacists' Association, Dr. Terry Babb, which helped gain early acceptance among pharmacists for the inclusion of EC in the collaborative practice agreements.[42] The pro-EC coalition worked to get the word out to the general public through media announcements and having a presence at various targeted venues such as the state fair and Alaska Women's Show.[43]

The persistence and success of the Alaska pro-Plan B coalition can be measured by the fact that 14 of the 19 communities with commercial pharmacies had been persuaded to get involved in the collaborative practice agreement. Similar to Washington State, the geography of service provision in Alaska is quite important and including EC in the direct pharmacist to client framework was a helpful step. The pharmacies were part of large retail chains, independent community-based shops, and a native medical center.[44] There were varied efforts by the pro-life movement in the state to require all women seeking Plan B to visit a doctor first, and one in 2003 to annul the collaborative practice agreement. Neither attempt was successful.

The third state in 2002 and fourth state of the nine to agree to include Plan B in the collaborative practice agreement was New Mexico. Just as Alaska was a pioneer in allowing nurses to become Plan B providers in its framework, New Mexico was innovative in developing a Web-based protocol. This protocol made New Mexico the first state to allow pharmacists to become the prescribers of Plan B at point of purchase by downloading the Web-based form.[45]

New Mexico built on the Washington state advocacy model of "relying heavily on physicians, particularly from the State Health Department" as well as those from the University of New Mexico and a broad group of pharmacists.[46] A helpful action by the University of Mexico's College of Pharmacy was to include EC provision in its required third-year curriculum so that all graduates have been trained in the protocol. Another important actor in this pro-choice network was the New Mexico Religious Coalition for Reproductive Choice that gave a grant to help train providers in four rural areas.[47] Barr Laboratories, by then the owner of Plan B, also provided funding for pharmacist training.

As it did in Washington, California, and Alaska, PATH helped to implement a pro-EC coalition at the state level. The New Mexico coalition was formed to aid in media strategies to increase awareness and education among the general population as well as policymakers and medical providers, and therefore to recruit and train more participants in the collaborative protocol. As usual, the coalition involved public health personnel and those from school-based clinics, doctors, pharmacists, and Planned Parenthood. At first, Dr. Diana Koster, medical director of Planned Parenthood, was the sole certified EC trainer in the state, but later, as in previous states, Don Drummond, the pharmacist trainer from Washington, was sent to New Mexico to perform the same job.[48] Media outreach was also important to targeted communities, as in California.[49]

Hawaii became the fifth state to add EC to its collaborative practice framework in 2003. However, a long, bureaucratic process followed, including the fact that the current Hawaii Administrative Rules process consists of 16 steps that include a lengthy review process by the attorney general's office, director's office, Legislative Reference Bureau, and scheduling public hearings, etc.[50] On November 13, 2003, the Hawaii Board of Pharmacy approved a change to the collaborative practice framework to include EC. By 2004, the rules still had not been accepted by the groups to which they had been sent, including the Hawaii Medical Association and the University of Hawaii's School of Medicine. Hawaii Women's Legislative Caucus publicly urged them to expedite the review process.[51]

By December 2004, the necessary approvals had been secured and Plan B distribution as part of the collaborative framework was put in place. There is still a fairly complex set of regulations in place, requiring any protocol changes to be sent to the state's Department of Commerce and Consumer Affairs. Another requirement that is supposed to help women is that if the EC-trained pharmacist named as the provider in the collaborative protocol is not on duty when a woman requests EC, the customer must be referred to another trained pharmacist.[52]

As in the other eight states, the state-based EC coalition was set up early, in 2002. One of the groups spearheading the initiative in Hawaii was the Healthy Mothers, Healthy Babies Initiative, a well-established public group in the state with a broad statewide steering committee. It had been established as a non-profit in 1992.[53] The framing by the latter group was particularly successful in stating that it aimed to reduce the teenage pregnancy rate. Other groups involved in the pro-EC network that PATH helped to establish included the proven successful formula combining representatives of the medical and pharmacists organizations, Department of Health, Planned Parenthood, and Kaiser Permanente, a large health maintenance organization in the state.[54] Undoubtedly, the presence of strongly pro-choice Republican governor Linda Lingle helped as did the networking with the Women's Legislative Caucus. Lingle was reelected to her second term as governor in 2006 and in 2007, Hawaii announced that it would extend Medicaid coverage to all Plan B provision, not just prescriptions.

Three New England states, Maine (2004), New Hampshire (2005), and Vermont (2007) followed the previous five early adopters in short order. The pro-EC networks in these states, part of the national framework organized by PATH, borrowed many of the successful strategies from previous states. The strategic influence of previous states was shown by the coalitions built between doctors' and pharmacists' organizations, public health representatives, Planned Parenthood representatives, and an increasingly prominent actor, the National Abortion Rights Action League (NARAL).

In Maine as in Alaska, the delegating authority does not have to be a physician. The state gives authority to nurses, nurse practitioners, certified nurse midwives, and physician assistants to enter the collaborative agreement. The process is that these providers can authorize the prescription and the pharmacist then downloads the protocol.[55] Maine was the first state to concurrently put into practice a general collaborative agreement and include EC in it.

The Emergency Contraception Access Campaign (ECAC) included the Family Planning Association of Maine, the Maine Health Access Foundation, and

Planned Parenthood of Northern New England (PPNNE) in addition to pharmacists, medical providers in all categories, and public health officials. The bill was first introduced in the 2003 legislative session and carried over into 2004. The 20-group ECAC coalition did a focused messaging strategy to legislators in the summer of 2003, talking about the risks of teenage pregnancy and the benefits to the usage of the safe and effective Plan B formula, particularly in the first 72 hours after intercourse. The Family Planning Association of Maine also developed fact sheets on the benefits of EC and PPNNE conducted educational sessions on college campuses. The law was passed in 2004 and took effect in July 2004. While pro-life groups, including the influential Catholic diocese, tried to add age restrictions to the bill, they were defeated. The Pharmacists' Association in Maine is responsible for developing and supervising the protocol for the collaborative agreements.[56]

As in Alaska and New Mexico, Maine's specific demographic issues included widely dispersed population centers across a large territory and a serious pharmacist shortage. Pharmacist Don Drummond was sent to Maine (and Vermont) to increase the pharmacist pool in the program, training over 200 pharmacists.[57]

The next state to add EC to a preexisting collaborative framework was New Hampshire, in June 2005. This state would not have been predicted as an early adopter, since it is a politically mixed bag with many libertarian Republicans from upstate and Democrats in the southern part of the state. The first bill to allow pharmacists to initiate EC provision (with a doctor's prescription on file) was introduced in 2001 but died in 2002. The broad proponent coalition was told that the bill died mainly since pharmacists had not been surveyed prior to its introduction and thus had not been involved in the bill's drafting.[58] In response, NARAL New Hampshire (NARAL-NH) began to work with PPNNE to build alliances "with pharmacists and physician groups and involved the newly reconstituted Reproductive Health Association, which has a broad membership of reproductive health professionals."[59] In addition, "PPNNE and NARAL-NH identified pharmacists and physician groups interested in working with local legislators to support EC. PPNNE also educated the press so they will not confuse EC with RU-486."[60] Finally, the pro-EC coalition interviewed pharmacists in summer 2002 and asked them whether they stocked EC and whether they had concerns about collaborative practice agreements concerning EC. NARAL-NH wrote follow-up letters thanking the pharmacists.[61]

The New Hampshire pharmacy access bill was reintroduced in 2004, and passed both legislative chambers despite unfavorable committee reports. The bill was vetoed by the first one-term governor since the 1920s, Republican Craig Benson, based on the familiar rhetoric of the George W. Bush administration that access to EC without prescription could encourage irresponsible sexual behavior and that there needed to be an age restriction in place. Proponents literally had to wait out the governor. Despite the fact that the New Hampshire governor is considered only second to that of Texas in terms of weakness, the legislature did not override the veto in 2004.[62]

After the Republican governor lost reelection in 2004, Democratic Governor Lynch signed the reintroduced EC access bill into law in June 2005, leaving it to the State Board of Pharmacists to implement the procedures. As in Maine, the strong pro-life lobby attempted to add an amendment to the legislation to effectively make the state's agreement mirror the national framework on age restrictions, and the attempted change was similarly defeated.

Massachusetts followed New Hampshire soon after in its addition of Plan B to the collaborative practice protocol, passing this law on December 14, 2005. The actions of then-governor Mitt Romney were similar to those of his New Hampshire neighbor, Craig Benson. Romney adopted the same incorrect language as Governor Benson and President George W. Bush had used, that "Plan B causes abortion in some instances."[63] In July 2005, Romney rushed back from his New Hampshire vacation to veto legislation that had been passed by an already veto-proof majority, and was thus overridden by the Massachusetts legislature a few months later. This incident undoubtedly made great political theater for those watching his preparations for his later run for the Republican presidential nomination. The incident does however negate his public statements in 2002 while running for Massachusetts governor that he favored EC. Massachusetts has been slow to implement the Plan B protocol through the collaborative practice agreements. A 2007 NARAL survey showed that only 3 of roughly half of the 500 pharmacists surveyed in the state were involved in an agreement.[64]

In Vermont, the addition of EC to the collaborative practice framework, including prescribers other than doctors, was signed into law by Republican governor James Douglas in March 2006. The Vermont Medical Society supported the bill and the Department of Health headed the process of public comment and review on the regulations.[65] In May 2007, after the implementation rules had been submitted to it, the Legislative Committee on Administrative Rules signed off on the framework and the state's pharmacy board approved the training for pharmacists.[66] As in many other states generally and the New England ones specifically, important parts of the pro-EC coalition included the Department of Health, Vermont Network against Domestic and Sexual Violence, and PPNNE. The Women's Health Center at the University of Vermont provided EC to university students.[67]

In terms of the relevant factors explaining the success of the nine states in adopting collaborative practice agreements between physicians (or other providers) and pharmacists to facilitate non-prescription EC access, some are covered by

Sidney Tarrow's political process model and aspects of historical institutionalism. With regard to the former, the pro-EC coalition acted quickly based on contacts in various states to implement networks that could be used to advocate for EC inclusion in collaborative practice agreements. The early implementation of alliances among pro-choice advocacy groups such as NARAL and Planned Parenthood; population think-tanks such as PATH, pharmacists, doctors, and nurses; and often state legislators fulfills Dorothy Stetson's description of the abortion policy triad, even though this particular scenario concerned an emergency-contraception triad.[68] Following Stetson's framework of women's pro-reproductive choice voices being transmitted through the state, voluntary sector and medical personnel enable us to see how important it was for pro-choice advocates to get to pharmacists and legislators before the other side did. This early access enabled the pro-choice coalition to become a proponent triad, in Stetson's terms, rather than shut out of policymaking as would be envisioned in Lowi's iron-triangle model.[69]

As shown throughout the discussion, sympathetic allies were important as per Tarrow's model, as was access to the state in the different states. Important allies included state pharmacists' professional organizations and the state-based American Medical Association, public health departments, Planned Parenthood or NARAL, and of course sympathetic women legislators. Helpful allies included Republican governors in at least two states. Most of the nine states had previous collaborative practice agreements, so one could argue that adding EC into them was a rather simple case of layering, as Jacob Hacker has described.[70] Alaska seems to have been a bit of an outlier since its collaborative practice agreement was only approved a year before EC was added to it. In terms of state size, professionalism of state legislature, and region of the country, fewer predictors line up in a linear fashion, showing that an unchanging historical institutionalist view of collaborative practice policy would not be the optimal explanation.

The models of discursive institutionalism formulated by Lombardo, Meier, and Verloo are relevant to framing the differences between the nine states that include Plan B provision in their collaborative practice agreements and the majority that do not.[71] From the standpoint of women's equality, the best possible type of discursive institutionalization of equality policy is that of stretching, which involves a "developing of a larger meaning that expands on its previous understanding in a given context."[72] Adding the provision of EC to the collaborative practice agreements of nine states fulfills the notion of stretching since this was a way to evade the restrictions placed on EC provision at the federal level. In those nine states, Plan B is not restricted by prescription status. Unhappily, it is also possible to point to the phenomenon of shrinking of gender equality in the EC example since the rest of the 45 states with collaborative practice agreements (36 of 45) do not include Plan B provision. Lombardo et al. defined shrinking as "reducing the meaning of the concept of gender equality down to a specific interpretation of the issue."[73] The national framework of Plan B provision as mostly lodged in the dualistic format of open access to those over 17 and prescription access to those under that age fits that definition.

STATE RESPONSES TO PHARMACIST
REFUSALS ON PRESCRIPTIONS

The first state to anticipate pharmacist refusal to fill prescriptions was Illinois. Governor Rod Blagojevich filed an emergency rule on April 1, 2005 to require pharmacies that "stock and dispense contraceptives to fill birth control prescriptions without delay."[74] This rule included Plan B. On April 18, 2005, he filed an action to make the emergency provision permanent, which gained the necessary approval by the legislature's Joint Committee on Administrative Rules on August 16, 2005.[75] The permanent rule also clarified a question in the previous standard, relating to whether any delay in filling a prescription was permissible. The new rule stated that pharmacists were required to fill all prescriptions without delay, meaning that "pharmacies should treat contraceptive prescription holders the same as other clients waiting for any other prescription."[76] By that point, pharmacist refusals to fill EC and other contraceptive prescriptions had been reported in several other states. These instances of refusal included "major drugstore chains, such as Walgreens, Osco, K-Mart, CVS, and Eckerd, as well as independently-owned drug stores."[77] In November 2005, Illinois suspended four Walgreen's pharmacists for declining to dispense EC. In addition to the new state law, the positive results from the Illinois case were that Wal-Mart began stocking EC there (the first state in which it did so), and CVS Corporation in May 2005 adopted the policy that its pharmacists must fill all lawful birth-control medication prescriptions.[78]

Women's pro-choice organizations also led a strong challenge to pharmacist refusals in Massachusetts. This challenge was based on the state law of 2005 and was mounted by Planned Parenthood and NARAL of Massachusetts and Jane Doe, Inc., a state-based organization that works with women who have been physically and sexually assaulted. This case became the second line of attack to force Wal-Mart to expand EC provision beyond the state of Illinois. Wal-Mart has been an interesting case study in this regard because while it was founded on and practices socially conservative beliefs, it is also the world's largest retailer (and pharmacy). Three plaintiffs, having been recruited by Planned Parenthood and NARAL, worked with a noted Massachusetts consumer protection attorney, Samuel Perkins. He filed the suit under the Consumer Protection Act, having won a settlement of 3.8 million dollars against Home Depot in 2002 for a consumer protection suit about pricing violations. Such were his clout, the strength of the Illinois precedent, and the new Massachusetts law that, after filing the suit against Wal-Mart on February 1, 2006 for having been denied EC, the women and their attorney saw a quick ruling by the Massachusetts Board of Pharmacy on February 14. At that time, the board ruled that Wal-Mart was required under the Massachusetts law to stock EC.[79] This marked the first time that Massachusetts had required a pharmacy to carry a particular drug.

Three days later, Connecticut followed Massachusetts's example. Comptroller Nancy Wyman asked Wal-Mart to stock EC there in its 20 pharmacies.[80] Attorney General Richard Blumenthal promised to work to ensure that the state insurance plan, covering 180,000 public employees and retirees, would not cover Wal-Mart prescriptions if their pharmacies did not dispense Plan B. Two days later, Wal-Mart changed its position, stating that all pharmacies in all states would stock Plan B.[81] The conscience guidelines for pharmacists opposed to EC from the American Pharmacists' Association specify that a dissenting pharmacist must refer the client to another pharmacist on duty or to another pharmacy where she can access the drug.[82]

Another example of political flip-flopping akin to that of Governor Romney was that of New York Governor George Pataki. Pataki had a 10-year record in New York as being not only pro-choice but also working for expanded access and increased public funding for abortions and contraceptives in New York.[83] When New York State was apparently his only political constituency, he took many brave stances on reproductive rights, often making him a nationwide minority, particularly for Republicans. These stances included signing legislation in 1995 that provided Medicaid funds for abortions for women of any age, and becoming the first governor to approve Medicaid coverage for RU-486 in 2001. In 2003, Governor Pataki signed the New York law to require emergency rooms to dispense EC for all women who had been raped.[84]

However, within two weeks of visiting Iowa (in July 2005) to test the presidential waters, Pataki announced that he would veto the EC bill that had recently passed, requiring EC to be available in pharmacies.[85] Even more interestingly, he claimed his objection was due to that of not having any provision in the bill about minors, taking a page out of New Hampshire governor Craig Benson's book. Pataki's claim seems especially inconsistent given that he previously went out on a limb to make abortion services and RU-486 that is an abortion drug, unlike Plan B, available to all via Medicaid funds. In New York, the NARAL state chapter ran an advertising blitz, urging Pataki not only to eye the Oval office but also the principles of New Yorkers as well.[86] Until 2012, there was no non-prescription provision of Plan B in New York, until New York City mandated it.

Currently, five states, those of Arkansas, Colorado, Maine, Mississippi, and Tennessee, have specific regulations allowing pharmacists to refuse to provide Plan B. Florida, Georgia, Illinois, and South Dakota have broad conscience clauses covering pharmacists.[87] The National Conference on State Legislatures lists 16 states as having passed legislation requiring hospitals or health-care facilities to provide information and/or EC to women who have been sexually assaulted.[88]

CONCLUSION

It has been shown that the U.S. system of diffused responsibility to 49 bicameral legislatures and a unicameral one has an enormous impact on women's ability to access the drugs and services needed to control their reproductive lives. The federalist framework of the United States, including health care and insurance provision plus the for-profit, private nature of the U.S. pharma industry, form enormous barriers to women's reproductive autonomy. Women in other countries may face access barriers of a federalist nature, but no other country houses the uniquely focused profit-making machine of U.S. pharma.

The theoretical foundations on which this analysis relies have been helpful in analyzing the barriers and alliances present in the efforts to make women's EC available OTC at the federal level. As shown, the dual regime of prescription-only access for women under 17 remains in 41 of the 50 states without the collaborative practice agreements concerning EC. In terms of historical institutionalism, the model of conversion is extremely important to showing the differences between the Clinton and George W. Bush administrations' FDA practices. Related to the conversion process was Baumgartner and Jones's punctuated equilibrium concerning the barriers faced to women at various times in Congress and the Executive since 1980. The increased representation of socially conservative Southern Republicans in those branches never boded well for women's reproductive autonomy. In turn, the punctuated equilibrium model shows a lack of state access for women (following Tarrow's theory) at particular critical points, such as in trying to persuade the Bush administration to consider and pass Barr's application for Plan B OTC status from 2003 to 2006. The historical institutionalist conversion model and the punctuated equilibrium one can implicate all three components of Tarrow's political opportunity structure. A generally unfriendly structure for reproductive rights present in the United States from 1980 onward, with the exception of the Executive branch under President Clinton, affected pro-choice access to the state, to alliances, and was obviously a product of changing political alignments.

In nine instances, in the collaborative practice agreement states the advocacy coalition for EC got out ahead of the opposition and got a positive infrastructure in place to implement EC access. This advocacy coalition included both older population research groups such as spin-offs from the Population Council and Population Action International, including PATH formed in the 1970s, and Planned Parenthood, as well as specific abortion-rights organizations such as NARAL. In terms of the policy triad discussed by Stetson, these groups worked with legislators, doctors, nurses, and pharmacists to add EC to the collaborative practice agreements. Access to the state was necessary in certain settings such as New Hampshire and Hawaii to push past a particularly unfriendly legislative or regulatory process. With respect to Hawaii, the 16 stages in its administrative rulemaking process could have formed an unwinnable barrier to proponents of the Plan B collaborative access agreement. Strong advocacy by Republican governor Linda Lingle and the Women's Legislative Caucus were certainly important. On the other hand, in many of the New England states where the Catholic church still exerts much political power and Church-affiliated health-care facilities are among the largest providers, the Republican governors of Maine and Massachusetts were able to stall but not prevent the inclusion of Plan B and all EC in collaborative practice agreements. In the nine states with collaborative practice frameworks, the pro-EC coalition was able to layer the drug onto the preexisting arrangements, following Streeck and Thelen's and Hacker's theories. The discussion of the different state environments shows that one cannot completely label the U.S. federalist structure as unfriendly to women. To supersede the diffuse structure with inertia against change, however, nearly superhuman efforts by powerful advocacy coalitions must happen. These superhuman efforts paid off in a number of states.

The creation of the Women's Capital Corporation and Gynetics showed the learning curve of the second-wave women's movement in the 1990s on reproductive issues. The strategic learning was necessary for women who had been figuratively hitting their heads against the wall for years in trying to interest large pharma companies in reproductive drugs. The answer was always the same, that such drugs were too risky to be allocated research time and funding. This was the case even as Searle, Johnson & Johnson, and other early doubters made fortunes from contraceptive patents. The new strategies of the pro-choice groups were modeled on and supported by the Population Council in particular, whose former executive members are on the boards of Gynuity and the International Consortium for Emergency Contraception. The learning displayed by the older groups in terms of forming newer, EC-specific groups also fulfills the criterion of forming positive alliances under Tarrow's formulation.

NOTES

1. Alicia Mundy, "Political Lobbying Drove FDA Process," *Wall Street Journal*, March 6, 2009, http://online.wsj.com/article/SB123629954783946701.html.

2. "FDA Chief Lester Crawford Resigns," *Fox News,* September 27, 2005, http://www.foxnews.com/story/0,2933,170285,00.html.

3. Wolfgang Streeck and Kathleen Thelen, "Introduction: Institutional Change in Advanced Political Economies" and Jacob Hacker, "Policy Drift: the Hidden Politics of US Welfare State Retrenchment," in *Beyond Continuity: Institutional Change in Advanced Political Economies,* eds. Wolfgang Streeck and Kathleen Thelen (Oxford: Oxford University Press, 2005), 1–39 and 40–82.

4. Michael A. Friedman, "FDA's Accomplishments and Proposals," *Testimony: U.S. FDA,* April 23, 1997, http://www.fda.gov/NewsEvents/Testimony/ucm114956.htm.

5. Emanuela Lombardo, Petra Meier, and Mieke Verloo, "Stretching and Bending Gender Equality: a Discursive Politics Approach," in *The Discursive Politics of Gender Equality: Stretching, Bending and Policymaking,* eds. Emanuela Lombardo, Petra Meier, and Mieke Verloo (London: Routledge, 2009), Chapter 1.

6. Charlotte Ellertson, "History and Efficacy of Emergency Contraception: Beyond Coca Cola," *Family Planning Perspectives* 28, no. 2 (March–April 1996): 44–48.

7. A. A. Haspels, "Emergency Contraception: A Review," *Contraception* 50, no. 2 (August 1994):101–8, cited in Ellertson, "History and Efficacy," 44.

8. Ellertson, "History and Efficacy," 44–45.

9. James Trussell, Charlotte Ellertson, and Felicia Stewart, "The Effectiveness of the Yuzpe Regimen of Emergency Contraception," *Family Planning Perspectives* 28, no. 2 (March–April 1996): 58–64, 97.

10. Ellertson, "History and Efficacy," 44.

11. A. A. Yuzpe et al., "Post Coital Contraception: A Pilot Study," *Journal of Reproductive Medicine* 13, no. 2 (August 1974): 53–58, cited in Ellertson, "History and Efficacy," 47.

12. Esteban Kesserii, Alfredo Larranaga, and Julio Parada, "Postcoital Contraception with D-Norgestrel," *Contraception* 7, no. 5 (1973): 367–79, cited in Ellertson, "History and Efficacy," 47.

13. Ellertson, "History and Efficacy," 44.

14. Premila W. Ashok, Catriona Stalder, Prabhath Wagaarachchi, Gillian M. Flett, Louise Melvin, and Allan Templeton, "A Randomised Study Comparing a Low Dose of Mifepristone and the Yuzpe Regimen for Emergency Contraception," *British Journal of Gynecology* 109, no. 5 (May 2002): 553–60.

15. World Health Organization, "Improving the Use and Supply of Medicines," *Essential Medicines Monitor* 34 (2005), http://apps.who.int/medicinedocs/index/assoc/s14078e/s14078e.pdf.

16. "EC in the News," *The Emergency Contraception Website,* http://ec.princeton.edu/news/index.html.

17. "Barr Pharmaceuticals, Inc. History," *Funding Universe,* http://www.fundinguniverse.com/company-histories/barr-pharmaceuticals-inc-history/.

18. "PREVENTM Emergency Contraceptive Kit—The First and Only Emergency Contraceptive Product—Approved by the FDA," *The Emergency Contraception Website,* http://ec.princeton.edu/news/preven.html.

19. "Barr Pharmaceuticals, Inc. History," *Funding Universe.*

20. *International Emergency Contraception Consortium,* www.cecinfo.org.

21. Michele Kort, "Denial by Delay," *Ms.* (Spring 2006): 12.

22. Kort, "Denial by Delay," 13.

23. Ibid., 12–13.

24. Cited in Kort, "Denial by Delay," 13.

25. Ibid.

26. Ibid.

27. "Timing of FDA Plan B Announcement Questioned," *The Medical News*, August 1, 2006, http://jurist.org.

28. Ibid.

29. Laura Blue, "Why the Plan B Debate Won't Go Away," *Time U.S.*, August 25, 2006, http://www.time.com/time/nation/article/0,8599,1333925,00.html.

30. News & Politics, "FDA to Allow Morning-After Pill Over the Counter for 17-Year Olds-CNN.com," *CNNHealthPolitics.com*, April 22, 2009, http://current.com.

31. Alesha E. Doan and Jean Calterone Williams, *The Politics of Virginity: Abstinence in Sex Education* (Westport, CT: Praeger, 2008), 14.

32. *PATH,* www.path.org.

33. "Sharing Public Health's 'Best-Kept Secret,'" *PATH,* http://www.path.org/projects/emergency-contraception-diverse-audiences.php.

34. Susan Kriemer, "Washington State Forges Physician-Pharmacist Partnering," *DOC News* 5, no. 1 (January 2008), http://docnews.diabetesjournals.org/content/5/1/12?patientinform-links=yes&legid=docnews;5/1/12.

35. "Emergency Contraception State Laws," *National Conference of State Legislatures (NCSL)*, July 2011, http://www.ncsl.org/issues-research/health/emergency-contraception-state-laws.aspx.

36. "Sharing Public Health's 'Best-Kept Secret,'" *PATH.*

37. Ibid. and "Pharmacy Access to Emergency Contraception," *National Women's Law Center,* April 22, 2012, http://www.nwlc.org/resource/pharmacy-access-emergency-contraception.

38. Ibid.

39. Donald Downing, "Pharmaceutical Care in Emergency Contraception," *Supplement to the Journal of the American Pharmaceutical Association* 42, no. 5 Suppl. 1 (September–October 2002): S38–S39, www.Go2Ec.org.

40. Ibid.

41. "State Access: Alaska," 2009, www.GO2EC.org.

42. Ibid.

43. Ibid.

44. Ibid.

45. "State Access: New Mexico," 2009, www.GO2EC.org.

46. Ibid.

47. Ibid.

48. Ibid.

49. Ibid.

50. "State Access: Hawaii," 2009, www.GO2EC.org.

51. Ibid.

52. Ibid.

53. Ibid.

54. Ibid.

55. "State Access: Maine," 2009, www.GO2EC.org.

56. Ibid.

57. Ibid.

58. "State Access: New Hampshire," 2009, www.GO2EC.org.

59. Ibid.

60. Ibid.

61. Ibid.

62. Anne Webber, "The Short, Strange Political Life of Craig Benson," *New Hampshire Wire*, January 5, 2005, http://www.wirenh.com/news-mainmenu-4/11-news-general/190-the-short-strange-political-life-of-craig-benson.html.

63. "State Access: Massachusetts," 2009, www.GO2EC.org.

64. Ibid.

65. "State Access: Vermont," 2009, www.GO2EC.org.

66. Ibid.

67. Ibid.

68. Dorothy Stetson, "Abortion Triads and Women's Rights in Russia, the United States, and France," in *Abortion Politics: Public Policy in Cross-Cultural Perspective*, eds. Marianne Githens and Dorothy Stetson (New York: Routledge, 1996), 97.

69. Theodore Lowi, *The End of Liberalism* (New York: Norton, 1969).

70. Jacob S. Hacker, "Policy Drift: The Hidden Politics of US Welfare State Retrenchment," in *Beyond Continuity* eds. Streeck and Thelen, 40–82.

71. Lombardo, Meier, and Verloo, "Stretching and Bending," Chapter 1.

72. Ibid., 5.

73. Ibid., 4.

74. "Governor Blagojevich Moves to Make Emergency Contraceptives Rule Permanent," *Illinois Government News Network*, April 18, 2005, http://www.illinois.gov/pressreleases/ShowPressRelease.cfm?SubjectID=1&RecNum=3862.

75. "Statement of Rachel Laser, NWLC Senior Counsel: NWLC Applauds Governor Blagojevich for Protecting Women's Access to Basic Health Care," *National Women's Law Center (NWLC)*, April 1, 2005, http://www.nwlc.org/sites/default/files/pdfs/4-1-05RLaser_ILPressStatement.pdf.

76. "Governor Blagojevich," *Illinois Government News Network*.

77. "Statement of Rachel Laser," *NWLC*.

78. Donna Goodison, "Holy Wars," *Boston Herald*, December 8, 2005, http://www.bostonherald.com.

79. Julie Jette, "State Board Leans on Wal-Mart," *The Patriot Ledger*, February 15, 2006, http://www.patriotledger.com.

80. "Comptroller Wants Wal-Marts to Stock Emergency Contraception," *Associated Press State and Local Wire*, February 17, 2006, http://w3.nexis.com.

81. Marcus Kabel, "Wal-Mart, in Reversal, to Stock Emergency Contraception Pill," *Associated Press State and Local Wire,* March 4, 2006, http://w3.nexis.com.

82. Goodison, "Holy Wars."

83. Brian McGuire, "Abortion-Rights Activists Vow to Make Pataki's Expected White House Bid an Uphill Battle," *The New York Sun,* August 2, 2005, http://www.nysun.com.

84. Ibid.

85. Ibid.

86. Ibid.

87. Guttmacher Institute, "Emergency Contraception: State Availability Chart," *www.guttmacher.org.*

88. "Emergency Contraception State Laws," *NCSL.* National Conference of State Legislatures www.ncsl.org

7

Reverse Lobbying for Gardasil

The Gardasil vaccine, manufactured by Merck for preventing four strains of human papillomavirus (HPV), has held a privileged position in the history of U.S. state and market treatment of women's reproductive drugs. Unlike the three other drugs discussed in this book, for which doctors, scientists, and the pro-choice women's community lobbied for decades, the Gardasil vaccine essentially sprang from a vacuum. A pressing, demonstrated need had not been established by the time the Food and Drug Administration (FDA) approved it in June 2006. Also, clinical trials had not yet been done on girls under the age of 11. This drug and Viagra for men, which was approved by the FDA in fewer than six months, are the two outliers in the typical history of state and market neglect to develop reproductive-related drugs. As has been shown earlier, while other actors typically have to cover the costs of research for these drugs up front, the pharma companies who license these drugs profit handsomely over the lifetime of their patents.

Gardasil covers four strands of the HPV, two of which have the strongest possibility to produce cervical, genital, and anal cancers. Seventy percent of such cancers are caused by HPV types 16 and 18. Gardasil was additionally engineered to target HPV strands 6 and 11 that can cause 90 percent of genital warts, although such warts do not lead to cancer. The Centers for Disease Control and Prevention

(CDC) states that genital HPV is the world's most common sexually transmitted infection, while a minority of the cases lead to cervical cancer.[1]

The bulk of the private- and public-sector actions around the approval and marketing of Gardasil had two goals. The first set of actions was to create a market for Gardasil that involved federal and state government actions never seen before or since regarding a drug oriented around sexuality. The second was to approve the U.S.-based vaccine prior to the competitor, Cervarix, which was coming up for FDA approval under the aegis of the British-based Burroughs-Wellcome company. The most prominent goal was to help Merck regain its position as a U.S.-based global pharma leader from 2005 onward. Originally a subsidiary of a German company, the U.S.-based company was formed when the German company's U.S.-based holdings were appropriated under World War I's Trading with the Enemy Act.[2] In 2005, Merck was facing millions of dollars in lawsuits from side effects related to Vioxx, and was also being pursued by the Internal Revenue Service for a 2-billion dollar amount owed.[3] The overriding imperative for Merck and the U.S. government was to find a new blockbuster for Merck.

Since the development of the Pap test in the 1940s, the incidence of cervical cancer in the United States and deaths from it has declined by 80 percent. As noted by Suraiya et al., the incidence of cervical cancer in the United States was also declining in the years before Gardasil was released. In the United States, Latinas and African American women tend to develop cervical cancer more than their white counterparts. While teenage Latinas and African Americans have higher rates of unplanned pregnancy than their white counterparts, it is women over 30 who get cervical cancer at higher rates than younger women. Cervical cancer is most often found in women who have either never had a Pap smear or who did not have one in the previous five years. Patterns in both the United States and the Global South (with the highest rates of cervical cancer) show the link between the diseases and women's lack of consistent access to reproductive health care. Padmanabhan et al. find that at least 80 percent of cervical cancer is in the Global South, with women in India accounting for 25 percent of the cases.[4] Globally, about 500,000 women develop cervical cancer each year and about 270,000 die.[5] Other countries where cervical cancer and deaths are rampant include sub-Saharan and Eastern Africa, Central America, and north and western Latin America including Venezuela, Colombia, Ecuador, Peru, and Bolivia.[6] The important issue to highlight at this point is that there was no health crisis regarding cervical cancer in the United States to which Merck was responding by fast-tracking the Gardasil vaccine in 2005–2006.

On a related note, the Global Alliance for Vaccines and Immunization (GAVI) website notes that 77 countries, the vast majority in Asia and Africa, are eligible for the vaccines GAVI provides. GAVI is funded and administered by the supranational health organizations' alliance created around the launch of the U.N. Millennium Development Goals in 2000. Funders and permanent seats on the GAVI Board are occupied by the Gates Foundation (which will fund HPV vaccines but nothing to do with abortion due to Melinda Gates's Roman Catholic religion), U.N. Children's Fund, the World Bank, and the WHO (World Health Organization).[7] Other seats go to world regions and a representative of the civil society sector, as well as to a representative of the vaccine industry from the Global North (industrialized countries) and Global South (industrializing countries). The alliance notes that it has "vaccinated 326 million children in the world's poorest countries" since it formed. In 2011, the GAVI Board approved the anti-HPV vaccines of Merck and GlaxoSmithKline (GSK) for use in their global vaccination program, noting the alliance's need to "work with the companies due to the high cost of the vaccine" that prevents the highest-incidence countries from purchasing the needed vaccine.[8] The website also stated that GAVI "hopes to begin inoculating girls by 2013, and to inoculate 28 million girls in the poorest countries by 2020." While the inclusion of HPV vaccines in the GAVI program is good given that at least 85 percent of deaths from cervical cancer are in the Global South, the lack of provision for women's comprehensive reproductive health over their lifetimes is a problem. Also the vaccine does not protect against any cervical, anal, or genital cancer already in process in one's body. Since the cancer is a very slow-moving one, it is likely that many already sexually active women will receive the vaccine in vain. Without regular Pap smears and follow-up, Gardasil and Cervarix will be at best expensive Band-Aids.

While it may seem uncharitable to put the actions of Merck and related supporters under a microscope, the critique lies in two parts of the equation. First, it is impossible to argue with the fact that Merck and the U.S. government starting in 2006 were "Johnny come latelies" to the cause of women's reproductive health, as were the U.N. agencies starting in 2000. Second, a corporation's or alliance's narrow emphasis on Gardasil prevents a focus on the underlying reasons for the prevalence of HPV and cervical cancer. A more comprehensive, integrated system of facilities, services, and insurance needs to be available in every country for women to have consistent access to reproductive health care. The Western European systems are the best at this, and Canada, the United States, and Australia are very much in the middle with inconsistent health-care services and laws, and insurance in the United States. The same factors are implicated as the relationship quickly spirals downward across other countries, particularly in Latin America and Asia, with sub-Saharan and Eastern Africa consistently at the bottom of the access list.[9] As has been demonstrated for the United States, a major factor in providing the relatively seamless network enjoyed by Western

Europe is that it does not have the same politics of for-profit pharma and the relationship to patent issues as in the United States. In general, in the Western European systems, there is a government-funded formulary governing the provision of prescription drugs. Once a decision has been made to include a drug on the formulary, whether still under patent or generic, it is then provided under the state-based health insurance system. The Western European countries tend to rely less on private insurers than the Anglo-American systems.[10] The rest of the countries, particularly in Latin America, Africa, and Asia, differ in the coverage available to those in the formal versus informal economies. Women are much more likely to be in the latter, and thus to have minimal coverage.

It is estimated that most sexually active U.S. women, up to 80 percent, become infected at some point with at least one of the many types of HPV. The CDC states that there are 40 strands of HPV that can cause genital or anal infection. According to one of the researchers who helped develop the vaccine, Dr. Diane Harper, most of the cases (up to 90%) resolve themselves within one year or two.[11] The American Cancer Society notes that cervical cancer is an extremely slow-developing cancer, with the majority of U.S. women diagnosed between the ages of 20 and 50. The society also notes that it is extremely rare to find cervical cancer in women under 20 and 20 percent of women diagnosed with it are affected when over 65.[12] The figures for incidence and death in 2012 are estimated by the American Cancer Society at just over 12,000 new cases of cancer and about 4000 deaths from it.

The low incidence of cervical cancer in the United States may be compared with the unmet contraceptive need for 15–44 year olds as shown in the unintended pregnancy rate of half of all pregnancies every year (3 million of the 6 million in the United States annually). Half of these pregnancies end in abortion.[13] While over half the states contain restrictions on the availability of abortion and contraception despite major Supreme Court decisions in the 1960s and 1970s, for example, more than half the states had introduced legislation to mandate Gardasil vaccination for schoolgirls within one year of its FDA approval.[14]

A related event concerning Merck's reach and lack of social conservatives' prurience when money is involved occurred in Canada, where incidence of and death from cervical cancer is about 1/10 of that in the United States (400 deaths per year). A former aide to Conservative Prime Minister Stephen Harper, Kenneth Boessenkool, became one of the chief lobbyists for Gardasil when Canadian subsidiary Merck Frosst hired Hill and Knowlton to lobby for the drug. Health Canada added Gardasil to its list of approved vaccines in July 2006, one month after the FDA had approved it. Also of note is that in 2007, the Canadian government announced a 300-million dollar program to pay for Gardasil for schoolgirls.[15] The Canadian education system is run differently from that of the United States and a blanket mandate for a certain age is not possible. Strong encouragement is a tool that can be used. The federal government used a financial inducement for Gardasil adoption, telling the provincial governments that they had to raise funds and participate in the program before the federal government's three-year funding allocation ended. Based on this urgency, 4 of the 10 provinces joined the program, making Gardasil a voluntary vaccination for public-school girls. As could be expected, the Catholic school systems of the provinces did not participate.

The federal government mandates of Stephen Harper since the Conservatives were first elected in 2006 have been viewed as socially conservative as the gubernatorial administrations of Rick Perry from 2001 to 2011. Given the well-publicized cuts to Planned Parenthood by the Canadian Conservative government since 2006 and its refusal to fund abortion services as part of Canadian foreign aid based on the 2010 G8 meetings held in Muskoka, Canada, its willingness to provide such funding for Gardasil is at the minimum inconsistent. Hill and Knowlton has been the chief global government-relations (lobbying) firm for both Merck and other big pharma firms, as well as for the WHO.[16] The Canadian government has also been a fairly prominent actor in the GAVI network. One avenue for that connection has been with the Grand Challenges program begun by the Gates Foundation, a chapter of which was formed in Canada (Toronto) in 2007, which participates in the global health solutions prioritized by the Gates Foundation. After the G8 Muskoka meetings in June 2010, the Harper government made an October 2010 announcement in which it promised 50 million dollars to GAVI "over the next five years . . . in addition to the $188 million Canada has provided to GAVI since 2001."[17] In 2007, a Merck press release noted that "as of the second quarter, Gardasil has been approved in 80 countries, many under fast-track or expedited review and launched in 59 of those countries."[18]

RELEVANT THEORETICAL FRAMEWORKS

Following from the previous case studies, the helpful frameworks for explaining the U.S. state (market and governments') different views and practices on Gardasil from their previous actions include historical and discursive institutionalism, the feminist interpretation of them used here, and Tarrow's political opportunity structure.[19] Clearly, Merck had access to the state. Unlike the RU-486 and Plan B cases, Merck was able to transcend the social conservative ambivalence about drugs related to women's sexuality that dominated Republican politics since 1980. Merck had many powerful alliances in the pharma industry, in the federal Bush administration, and in the Texas Perry administration. The company used these alliances successfully to create a public sense of urgency around the need for anti–cervical cancer vaccinations in the United States, even though the vast majority of cases occurred in the Global South. Probably not surprisingly, progressive women were convinced that Gardasil was a much-needed vaccine in the United States and that it was an effort worth supporting.

In certain ways the Merck-Gardasil case study shows the persistence of Lowi's iron-triangle framework and how the reproductive policy triad described by Stetson can at times be used against women's interests.[20] The triangle of Merck, politicians, and the carefully selected anti-cancer and women's legislative groups was controlled by Merck in its quest to find a quick, profitable replacement for Vioxx. Vioxx was removed from the global market in 2005. On the other hand, doctors were not as strongly in favor of Gardasil as they had been for Plan B and thus they cannot be said to have formed a strong part of the reproductive policy triad in this instance. Many physicians expressed skepticism as to whether Gardasil could fulfill all the promises made by Merck.

In terms of feminist discursive institutionalism, the Gardasil case can be linked to Lombardo et al.'s concepts of bending and shrinking. Bending of gender equality occurs when a policy gets changed so that gender equality is no longer the goal.[21] It is easy to see this happening with respect to Gardasil, where the public rhetoric was framed as protecting young girls but the underlying reality was that Merck needed a blockbuster drug as fast as possible. The process of shrinking a policy frame, according to Lombardo et al., occurs when the meaning of a policy is confined to a specific interpretation of the issue.[22] The Gardasil issue was simultaneously shrunk to the meaning of protecting girls, and bent because it was much more related to protecting Merck's fortunes than young women.

Historical institutionalist understandings can also be related to this feminist-based study. Since the marketing of Gardasil, both pre– and post–FDA approval, was centered around helping Merck more than U.S. women, we can see a combination of the Streeck and Thelen layering and drift at work. Drift is described by Hacker as a consistently negative phenomenon, whereby an agency or policy program loses its accountability to its initial constituency.[23] Hacker characterizes drift as a process of preventing institutions from adapting to social change. Of course, his characterization of drift is consistent with the way Baumgartner and Jones describe the lead-up to a policy punctuation and to Burnham's theory of the forces driving party realignments.[24] The three models share in common the idea that social circumstances change faster than political institutions can adapt to them. Burnham and Baumgartner and Jones envision a profound political rupture in response to the mismatch. Streeck and Thelen speak of conversion in this regard. This model is used when institutions are directed to new goals, functions, or purposes.[25] Following from previous discussion, we know that conversion of the policy subsystem responsible for women's and children's health in the Department of Health and Human Services (HHS) and the FDA as part of it began in 1980 under Ronald Reagan and flowered fully under the George W. Bush presidency. The conversion of the policy subsystem was itself based on the Republican realignment starting in 1980. The 1980 realignment yielded a policy punctuation on women's reproductive health, following the Baumgartner and Jones model, which then enabled a conversion of the policy subsystem.

The most important point of relating historical institutionalist theories to this particular feminist study is that the policy punctuation and related conversion of the women's reproductive health structures and discourse after 1980 brought about both drift in this policy subsystem and a negative form of layering. The negative form of layering is seen in the Gardasil example, where a new drug was made available very quickly, but not for feminist purposes. The entire process of marketing Gardasil and related vaccination programs was driven by male pharma execs and legislators to boost Merck's profits. Women's voices in this scenario were manipulated by the male actors to support the claim and layer a feminist voice onto the Gardasil project. In the larger historical context, the layering of Gardasil onto the history of the U.S. public and private sectors' interference with developing and marketing women's reproductive drugs might have made it appear that the usual male and financial bias of the drug policy system in the United States had changed. This analysis shows why that optimism is unwarranted, and how Gardasil proves the rule.

HISTORY OF THE VACCINE

The link between HPV and genital and cervical cancers was first discovered in Germany in the 1980s. As described by the in-house instrument of the peak organization of the U.S. pharma lobby (Pharmaceutical Researchers and Manufacturers of America, PhRMA), the Innovation.org newsletter, "in the 1970s and 1980s, Harald zur Hausen of Germany established a link between HPV and cervical cancer, work that took him ten years to complete and won him a Nobel prize just last year. Subsequent research by the Australian Ian Frazer demonstrated the potential of synthesizing virus-like particles (VLPs) from recombinantly expressed HPV capsid protein to resemble actual viral particles."[26] The marvel of this discovery, according to PhRMA, was that this research demonstrated the first convincing link between a virus and cancer.

According to Padmanabhan et al., the vaccine was first created at the National Cancer Institute (part of the National Institutes of Health [NIH], which is part of the U.S. HHS), working with the University of Rochester, Georgetown University, and the University of Queensland (Australia). The companies MedImmune, Merck, and GSK then developed proprietary interests in the vaccines and sponsored clinical trials to prove safety and efficacy.[27] Mark Blaxill, an autism and anti-vaccine activist and author, states that the NIH is the world's single largest sponsor of biological research. He has also written that two National Cancer Institute scientists, Douglas Lowy and John Schiller, invented the virus-like particle technology used in the Gardasil vaccine. NIH licensed the technology to both Merck and GSK.[28]

Blaxill also noted that "Gardasil is perhaps the leading example of a new form of unconstrained government self-dealing, in arrangements whereby DHHS can transfer technology to pharmaceutical partners, simultaneously both approve and protect their partners' technology licenses while also taking a cut of the profits." Blaxill stated that this particular public–private partnership program started at HHS in 2005 and that "DHHS agencies have become more aggressive about pursuing them." Finally, Blaxill notes that "the potential for conflict of interest exists any time the NIH and NIH staff engage with non-Federal entities to achieve mutual goals."[29]

There were many public- and private-sector fingers in the discovery pie, as Padmanabhan et al. show through the number of patents granted. As of 2010, they found that 81 U.S. patents had been granted for HPV vaccines. Of those 81, non-profits owned 20 patents, for-profits owned 20, and for- and non-profit entities jointly owned 6. They stated that "Merck owns the most patents, 24, followed by GSK and the US government, who own eight patents each."[30]

Given the combined financial interest of Merck and the U.S. government in pushing ahead with a new blockbuster, Gardasil was given an expedited review by the FDA. The initial drug application was submitted December 5, 2005, and on May 18, 2006, the advisory committee voted unanimously to approve it. FDA approval was publicly announced on June 8, 2006, to be administered to girls and women from 9–26 years old.[31] The speed with which this vaccine was approved can only be compared with Viagra, which was also given the green light within six months. Both Gardasil and Viagra were sped through approvals by the FDA under the second George W. Bush administration, while EC (Plan B) approval was dragged out from 2000 until 2006.[32] Interestingly but probably coincidentally, the Bush administration finally capitulated at least on allowing Plan B to be sold over the counter for those 18 and under in August 2006, a few months after Gardasil was released.

Strangely, British-owned GSK faced more than a two-year delay of trials required by the FDA. This outcome was odd given that the technology for both vaccines was developed at the same time at NIH and that the GSK-licensed vaccine only covered two HPV strands, a vaccine for which had already been approved by the FDA. Bearing out the pattern noted for U.S.- versus foreign-owned companies, GSK faced more than a two-year FDA review and clinical trials in between its new drug application and final approval.[33] It has been noted that "the FDA required more long-term trials of Cervarix than it did of Gardasil."[34] GSK states that Cervarix is a better vaccine given that its propriety adjuvant (additive) AS04 increases the potency of the vaccine. The two vaccines, the quadrivalent HPV4 Gardisil and bivalent HPV2 Cervarix, are said to give five years of protection against the four or two strands targeted. These vaccines will neither affect the existing HPV in the body nor stop precancerous or cancerous changes. It is also known that there can be a 10-year period for women who are infected with HPV to develop fully manifested cervical cancer.

As summarized by Emma Hitt, Gardasil was approved for routine use among females aged 9–26 (with the target populations typically at 11–12 years of age) in 2006.[35] This approval included the FDA and also the CDC's Advisory Committee on Immunization Practices (ACIP), with both located in HHS. On October 16, 2009, a soft recommendation by ACIP (not a general routine recommendation) was made for Gardasil to be given to boys and men from ages 9 to 26. The target range was boys from 11 to 12 years of age, with catch-up vaccines within the general age range permitted. Cervarix was also approved by the FDA on that date and added to ACIP's list of recommended vaccines, but only for 10–25-year-old girls and women (as opposed to Gardasil's 9–26-year age range). Cervarix has also had the catch-up provision added into ACIP's recommendation. Cervarix has never been approved for boys and men. Finally, on October 25, 2011, ACIP announced its strong recommendation for routine vaccinations of men and boys 9–26 years of age with Gardasil, the quadrivalent vaccine.[36] Where men and boys are concerned, Gardasil and Merck hold the entire U.S. market share.

The denoting of a vaccine as approved by ACIP holds clear implications for payment. As Alexandra Stewart has noted,

An ACIP (Advisory Committee for Immunization Practices) recommendation triggers government and private programs that are designed to increase access to vaccines among appropriate populations. Public programs that ensure the availability of vaccines include the Vaccines for Children Program, Medicaid, 317 grant programs, and state and local delivery mechanisms. Private-market health insurance plans may rely on ACIP recommendations to make coverage decisions. Finally, states often modify the list of vaccines that are required for school entry to comply with administration schedules developed by ACIP.[37]

While Gardasil was still under review, the Merck company spent 841,000 dollars on Internet ads alone promoting the drug during the first quarter of 2006.

This may be compared against total ad spending by U.S. pharma companies during 2005 of 4.8 billion dollars.[38] As *Bloomberg News* noted, it was an extremely unusual occurrence to advertise drugs before FDA approval. The same article quoted Richard Haupt, executive director of medical affairs in Merck's vaccine division as stating that Merck had "invested in public affairs and consumer education more than we've done for any vaccine in the past."[39] It is clear that much was at stake for Merck with this drug, needing a blockbuster at the time, and the U.S. government headed by George W. Bush and his HHS secretaries, first former governor Tommy Thompson (R-WI) and then former governor Michael Leavitt (R-UT) understood that. The evidence lies in the expedited review given to Gardasil even when studies were not complete, and forcing GSK to continue them.

THE POLITICS OF THE GARDASIL VACCINE MANDATE

Mandating the drug for various categories was a sure way to get people to pay for the drug. As it stands, those without insurance coverage for it typically do not complete the 375-dollar series of three vaccines. Based on the 1996 Illegal Immigration Reform and Immigrant Responsibility Act, another avenue was found to help Merck through the legislation's vaccination requirement.[40] The 1996 act included the typically contagious diseases of mumps, measles, rubella, polio, tetanus and diphtheria toxoids, pertussis and influenza type B, and hepatitis B. Just after the FDA approved Gardasil in 2006 and Cervarix in 2009, the CDC added these vaccines to the list of visa requirements. Also, based on viewing HPV as the most highly contagious sexually transmitted microbe, the U.S. Department of Defense added it to its highly recommended list of vaccines. Of course the irony should not be missed that under the Bush administration, female military personnel and spouses could not access abortions on military bases but could get their Gardasil shots there.

Texas governor Rick Perry was the first to mandate Gardasil vaccination for girls. Observers believe that his odd enthusiasm for the vaccine given his oft-stated social conservative views was due to two sources. The first was his former chief of staff Michael Toomey, who was a Merck lobbyist in 2007. The second reason for the Governor's support came from his then chief of staff Deirdre Delisi, whose mother in law was the state chair for Women in Government Foundation (WIG), a group co-opted by Merck, as will be discussed. Newspaper accounts of Texas politics refer to the pay-to-play culture, particularly under the long-standing governorship of Rick Perry since 2001. Perry started his career as a state Democratic House Representative and then, like others including former U.S. senator Jesse Helms and President Ronald Reagan, switched party labels to get elected to higher office.

The pay-to-play culture in Texas has involved an unusually tight relationship between business lobbyists and politicians. One example was under the George W. Bush governorship starting in 1996 when funds were made available for abstinence-based programs in the state. That same year, Congress passed the Personal Responsibility and Work Opportunity Reconciliation Act (PROWRA), which included funding for abstinence-based education programs, including funds that could be given to state anti-choice crisis pregnancy centers. These centers are framed by reproductive rights activists as anti-choice since their goal is to convince women not to have abortions. As is now known, the funding for abstinence-based education really took off under the George W. Bush presidency. However, as Siecus states that at best, the cumulative impact of the Title V expenditures was about 2 billion dollars by the time President Bush left office in 2009, as opposed to the 1 billion plus dollars per year raised by mandating Gardasil shots in the United States.[41]

Merck's U.S.-based lobbying was not only in the hands of its own personnel, including Michael Toomey in Texas, but also in the firms of Edelman and Cohn & Wolfe/GCI.[42] Michael Toomey, a former legislator, chief of staff to two governors including Rick Perry from 2002 to 2004 and then a member of the Texas Lobby Group, has been a crucial supporter of Perry's.[43] In 2007, Toomey was Merck's sole lobbyist in Texas and charged with getting the mandate for Gardasil. On February 2, 2007, Governor Perry obliged, issuing an executive order mandating vaccinations for 11- and 12-year-old schoolgirls (with a parental opt-out clause).[44] Since there were 165,000 girls in this universe annually, it was estimated that the Texas program alone could bring in 55–60 million dollars per year.[45] This figure could also expand through the federally-funded Texas Vaccines for Children program (covering ages 9–18), as well as Medicaid coverage for women aged 19–21.[46] Governor Perry's willingness to allow Gardasil to be funded through Medicaid seems slightly contradictory to the Texas policy of only allowing Medicaid funding for abortions in the extreme cases of rape, incest, or life endangerment.[47] The paradox of these policies is that they both seem to recognize the existence of sex between men and women. However, only the Gardasil approval could be traced to a profit incentive.

The Texas legislature disagreed with Perry's mandate, and overturned it in three months. The financial link remained between Michael Toomey, Merck, Governor (and then Republican nominee candidate) Perry, and the national Republican Governors' Association (RGA), which Perry headed from 2008 to 2011. While candidate Perry dismissed presidential debate opponents' mention of the Merck payments to him by claiming that "he could not be bought for 5,000" (the amount of a one-time contribution), the Merck interest in Perry was far larger. While Merck gave Perry the stated 5000 dollar amount in October

2006, it also gave him a total of 28,500 dollars during his 11-year governorship of Texas since 2001 and 377,500 dollars to the RGA while Perry headed it from 2008 to 2011.[48] As noted by *Washington Post* journalist Dan Eggen, the RGA "ranked among Perry's largest donors, giving him at least $4 million since 2007."[49]

Other general examples of the Perry–Toomey financial links include the following. As the *New York Times* noted in August 2011, the Governor's Office, through an economic development fund it controlled, gave 3 million dollars to G-Con, a pharma start-up company founded by large Democratic donor John McHale. McHale has been noted to have given at least 100,000 dollars directly to Governor Perry for his reelection efforts. Similarly, "at least two other executives with connections to the firm had given Mr. Perry tens of thousands of dollars."[50] The same article stated that, "Mr. Perry has raised at least $17 million from more than 900 appointees or their spouses, roughly one dollar out of every five that he has raised as governor." Another quote about Toomey's enforcement capabilities is the following:

> (former State Representative Tommy) Merritt said Toomey summoned him to his House office in 2004 and warned that he could "call the six richest people in Texas and take me out" unless Merritt supported the re-election of the sitting House speaker and Perry ally, Tom Craddick. "I did what he asked," Merritt said. The lawmaker said he got something in return: Perry's endorsement for his House seat.[51]

Toomey's clients received 2 billion dollars from the Texas government between 2008 and 2011. Toomey was also the chair of the super political action committee (PAC) Make Us Great Again, with a reputed 50-million-dollar budget as of October 2011.[52] Super PACs made an entrance into the 2012 presidential nominating campaigns in the wake of the noted *Citizens' United vs. FEC* U.S. Supreme Court decision of January 2010, overturning previous Federal Election Act restrictions on electioneering ads aired by unions, corporations, or nonprofits. The same pretense at non-coordination between candidate and super PAC is continued, and maintaining that is sufficient for a super PAC to raise and spend unlimited amounts in favor of their candidates.

MERCK'S CREATION OF A WOMEN'S LOBBY FOR GARDASIL

Merck hit the ground running in several attempts to create publicity for itself and the link between HPV and cervical cancer in public awareness before the FDA approved Gardasil in June 2006. Chronologically, the earliest effort started in 2005 and was called Make the Connection, run by a previously existing non-profit group called the Cancer Research and Prevention Fund (CRPF). In its public vaccine promotion from 2005 to 2007, Merck typically co-opted an existing infrastructure. While the groups ultimately co-opted by Merck were initially formed for sincere reasons, such as anti-cancer activism or progressive politics by women state legislators, their actions were judged in the final analysis by how rich Merck became from Gardasil.

The CRPF was formed in 1985 by a young woman named Carolyn Aldige after her father died from cancer.[53] By 2006, CRPF was bringing in hundreds of thousands of dollars per year from many pharma firms, including the sector's peak organization lobby firm, PhRMA. The firms included Merck, GSK, Pfizer, Roche, Eli Lilly, and Sanofi-Aventis. As Siers-Poisson has noted, "partnering with non-profits, especially non-profits that appear to have patients' health and women's issues as their primary concerns, helped Merck reach audiences that may have rightly been suspicious of the motivations of a pharmaceutical company."[54] In fact, many of the same pharma companies appear as clients of Hill & Knowlton and Edelman used in the U.S. lobby effort for Gardasil.

Another partner of Merck's in the 2005 Make the Connection campaign was a non-profit known as the Step Up Women's Network. According to the network's website (www.suwn.org), it was formed by a woman named Kaye P. Kramer in 1998 by inviting 30 of her friends over to discuss the fact her mother had been diagnosed with breast cancer. It is now described as a "non-profit membership organization dedicated to connecting and advancing girls and women," and lists many heavy-hitting U.S. and global firms including Nestle, Gillette, CBS, and Bayer.[55] As a former celebrity agent and furniture store owner, Kaye Kramer has been well-positioned to draw in Hollywood stars to her efforts to help disadvantaged girls and women, which probably made this group attractive to Merck for the Make the Connection push. As noted by Siers-Poisson, the idea was to educate the public to make the connection between HPV and cancer (and of course Merck) by using the standard formula of a celebrity, a medical professional, and an opportunity for attendees to bead their own Make the Connection bracelets. Such bracelets were then worn by prominent stars on TV and in print ads.

As Siers-Poisson has written, Make the Connection amped up in volume to "Make a Commitment," which continued the high-profile events around the country at which celebrities appeared and talked to girls and women. The campaign also involved placing many ads on the TV, Internet, and in women's and girls' magazines. A related strategy was that where women and girls were exhorted to tell someone about the dangers of HPV. While the drug itself could not be named in ads before FDA approval, the Merck logo and name were prominently placed. In this Tell Someone strategy, the ads' actors wore white T-shirts emblazoned with the logo and appeared shocked that there could be millions of women walking around with a form of HPV and not know it.[56] Of course, that is still true, since the vaccines protect at best against only four HPV strands and we know that the majority of sexually active people contract at least some form of HPV during their lives.

After the vaccine was approved in June 2006 and was added to the CDC's list of recommended immunizations, Merck kept on lobbying, both in the United States and around the world. A few months after FDA approval, in November 2006, Merck launched its direct-to-consumer advertising, as if the previous campaigns had somehow seemed indirect. The same media types were used, with the new slogan "One Less" being promoted.[57]

WOMEN IN GOVERNMENT

However blatant the celebrity- and ordinary-girl advertisements were, they were well-matched by Merck's (and other pharma companies') instrumental relationship with the WIG, formed in 1988. While both WIG and the National Conference of State Legislatures (NCSL) are bipartisan, the similarities end there. In its board and funding, the WIG is the exact opposite of the publicly-funded NCSL that is comprised of state legislators. The NCSL does not accept corporate donations and does not allow corporate representatives to sit on its board. It is a publicly-funded lobby group for state legislators to represent their interests to the national government.[58] While the NCSL does have a foundation that works closely with corporate America and accepts corporate contributions, WIG exists solely as a foundation funded by the private sector (heavily from health care and pharma).[59] The WIG which describes itself as a forum where women state legislators can meet and discuss innovative solutions to policy challenges. Siers-Poisson listed some of the funders of WIG as, in addition to Merck and GSK, Novartis, Eli Lilly, AstraZeneca, Bayer Healthcare, Pfizer, Bristol-Myers Squibb (both the company and their foundation), and PhRMA, the largest national pharma lobby representing close to 50 corporations in 2007.[60] The other company that remained a constant over time on WIG's funding list, stated Siers-Poisson in addition to Merck and GSK, was Digene, which created the only FDA-approved HPV test. In 2007, the German corporation Qiagen bought Digene (and thus the rights to the HPV test) in order to become a "market and technology leader in molecular diagnostics."[61]

As Siers-Poisson noted, WIG members were heavily involved in trying to convince colleagues in 23 states by 2007 to put forth vaccine mandates or mandates with the common medical and religious parental opt-out provisions.[62] In many states, a fine line was drawn (and in some cases crossed) whereby legislators became the mouthpieces of Merck. On one hand, it is easy to understand that based on the often presented, highly selective evidence doled out by the company in the first few years of Gardasil's existence that women would have felt an imperative to share the news of the vaccine with friends and colleagues. After all, it was the first vaccine against cancer. On the other, some women legislators became extremely disenchanted with the pro-Merck tilt of the effort and began to question the validity of the evidence used. For example, at a WIG Annual State Directors' Conference in 2007, two Maine Democratic state legislators, Marilyn Canavan and Andrea Boland reported becoming uncomfortable with the laser-like focus on promoting Gardasil. They reported that when they asked questions, the response was to ask whether they wanted their daughter to die from cancer.[63] They also reported that when asking about the priorities for the next year, they were told to "wait to see who the funders are." These state legislators felt like they were the dogs being wagged by the Merck tail, and Canavan resigned from WIG shortly thereafter. It is likely that the majority of WIG members involved in the fight against HPV and to introduce vaccine-enabling legislation thought they were doing a service to the U.S. population. For example, one leader of the effort in Illinois, Debbie Halvorson, Democratic majority leader of the Illinois senate, had required a hysterectomy due to HPV infection. While she worked hard to get legislation introduced for Gardasil there, she also believed that Merck was pushing the whole effort too hard and it "seemed like Merck was pushing our buttons."[64]

According to the CDC, all states allow vaccine refusal for evidence that adverse medical conditions would result if a child/adult got the required vaccine. Some states allow this refusal for permanent disability only, some for temporary as well. The District of Columbia and 47 states allow refusals for religious belief, and 18 states allow refusals based on the parents' philosophical views.[65] The three mandates of 2007 passed in Texas, Virginia, and the District of Columbia all had exemptions included. During the same legislative session, at least 20 other state assemblies were considering some form of bills recommending the vaccine or at least public education about it. By February 2007, it appeared that Merck had become too pushy and so it announced it was discontinuing its efforts in the states. One could speculate that it felt it could afford to do so, given that its 2007 annual report extolled the fact that it had launched the vaccine in 59 of the 80 countries where it had been approved. By that point, Merck had also appeared prominently on the radar screens of social conservative organizations that were venting their wrath on the sexually permissive practice of vaccinating young women. While these groups such as Focus on the Family and women's groups Eagle Forum and Concerned Women for America had little if any persuasive power over Merck, they were making the state climate uncomfortable in some legislatures. Also, Merck did not want to jeopardize its new golden goose egg that was to lift it out of the Vioxx doldrums. On the other hand, Merck is a member of the American Legislative Exchange Council that announced in April 2007 that it was forming an HHS task force to study state vaccine mandates. In July 2011, the NCSL reported that "legislators in at least 41 states and DC have introduced legislation to require, fund or educate the public about the HPV vaccine and at least 20 states have enacted this legislation."[66]

The same report listed certain states as having announced their participation in the federal-state vaccination funding programs since 2006, including New Hampshire, which provides the vaccine free to girls under 18. In 2007, the state reported that it had distributed more than 14,000 doses. South Dakota engaged in a similar plan in January 2007, contributing 1.7 million dollars to the federal effort there of 7.5 million dollars, and by May 2007 reported distributing more than 20,000 doses to girls and women. The Washington state legislature approved 10 million dollars to cover 94,000 girls from 2011 to 2013. [67] In California in October 2011, Governor Jerry Brown signed a Gardasil mandate for 12-year-old boys and girls into law. While the specific law does not contain exemptions, California does allow medical, religious, and philosophical exemptions for vaccines. This is an issue that may well come before the courts.

CONCLUSION

In direct contradiction to the three earlier case studies, the Gardasil vaccine was based on no proven medical need at the time it was introduced by Merck. Where it was most needed, it was not available and is only slowly becoming available through the GAVI Alliance. While Merck has made its desired 1 billion dollars annual minimum from Gardasil, the vaccine has, to quote Judith Siers-Poisson, "not been the shot in the arm Merck hoped for." In between the heady advertising push of 2006–2007 and 2012, people became more educated about the limitations of the vaccine and the ratio of adverse effects. The national Vaccine and Adverse Effects Reporting System that works with both FDA and CDC in the HHS in 2009 compared reports of side effects from Gardasil with those from Menactra, the vaccine against meningitis approved in 2005. On nearly every type of criterion, the Gardasil vaccine outweighed the Menactra one for problematic events: more than 10,000 total reports for Gardasil as opposed to 4400+ for Menactra, 152 life-threatening incidences for Gardasil versus 52 for Menactra, 5021 versus 1667 emergency room visits, 458 versus 268 hospitalizations, 2017 versus 393 instances of did not recover, 261 versus 29 reports of becoming disabled from the respective vaccines, and 29 vs. 6 deaths.[68] These figures certainly warrant a rethinking of how much to use the vaccine, and indeed the report concluded with the statement that "immediate action should be taken now by federal health to protect recipients of Gardasil from injury and death." Clearly, such action was not taken, since in October 2009, after the report was released, the FDA approved Gardasil for boys and men and made an even stronger recommendation for routine shots for boys and men in the 9–26 age range in 2011. It also promoted catch-up Gardasil shots for all populations.

What the example of Gardasil shows is the following. First, the gendered historical institutionalist studies are on target in showing that the pharma system in the United States has traditionally been and still is dominated by concerns that exclude the reproductive health of women. Given the prevalence of cervical cancer in the Global South, this lack of attention is even worse outside the United States. Second, it shows that when the time is right (i.e., a drug company needs massive infusions of cash), the planets can be moved to expedite the approval of a vaccine for which women did not lobby. Finally, the example continues to prove that the majority of Americans and consumers, women, still do not have an equal place at the public- and private-sector tables where decisions about their reproductive health are taken.

NOTES

1. "Genital HPV Infection: Fact Sheet," *Centers for Disease Control and Prevention (CDC)*, http://www.cdc.gov/std/hpv/stdfact-hpv.htm/.

2. Edward Graham and David Marchick, *US National Security and Foreign Direct Investment* (Washington, DC: Institute of International Economics, 2006).

3. Judith Siers-Poisson, "Setting the Stage: Part One in a Series on the Politics and PR of Cervical Cancer," *PR Watch*, June 26, 2007, http://prwatch.org/node/6186.

4. Swathi Padmanabhan, Tahir Amin, Bhavan Sampat, Robert Cook-Deegan, and Subhashini Chandrasekharan, "Intellectual Property, Technology Transfer and Developing Country Manufacture of Low-Cost HPV Vaccines: A Case Study of India," *Nature Biotechnology* 28, no. 7 (July 2010): 671–78.

5. "Eliminating Cervical Cancer," QIAGENcares, January 1, 2010, http://www.qiagen.com/about/whoweare/qiagencares/creating-a-world-free-from-cervical-cancer.pdf.

6. Ibid.

7. *GAVI Alliance*, http://www.gavialliance.org/.

8. "GAVI Recognized for Work to Accelerate Introduction of HPV Vaccines in Developing Countries," *GAVI Alliance*, March 8, 2012, http://www.gavialliance.org/library/news/press-releases/2012/gavi-recognised-hpv-vaccines-in-developing-countries/.

9. "Fact Sheet: Facts on Induced Abortion Worldwide," *Guttmacher Institute*, January 2012, http://www.guttmacher.org/pubs/fb_IAW.html.

10. Scott L. Greer and Bert Vanhercke, "The Hard Politics of Soft Law: The Case of Health," in *Health Systems Governance in Europe: The Role of European Union Law and Policy,* eds. Mossialos, Elias, et al. (Cambridge: Cambridge University Press, 2010), 186–230, esp. 207–12.

11. Siers-Poisson, "Setting the Stage," June 2007.

12. "Cervical Cancer," *American Cancer Society,* http://www.cancer.org/Cancer/CervicalCancer/index.

13. "Fact Sheet: Facts on Induced Abortion in the United States," *Guttmacher Institute,* August 2011, http://www.guttmacher.org/pubs/fb_induced_abortion.html/.

14. Judith Siers-Poisson, "The Gardasil HPV Vaccine: Not the Shot in the Arm Merck Hoped For," *PR Watch,* September 16, 2008, http://www.prwatch.org/news/2008/09/7748/gardasil-hpv-vaccine-not-shot-arm-merck-hoped.

15. Tanya Talaga, "Lobbyists Boosted Vaccine Program," *Toronto Star,* August 16, 2007, http://www.thestar.com/news/article/246824--lobbyists-boosted-vaccine-program.

16. "Ken Boessenkool, Merck, and the Conserva-Liberal Flip Flop," *Canadian Gardasil Awareness Network,* October 23, 2011, http://www.canadiangardasilawarenessnetwork.com/1/post/2011/10/ken-boessenkool-merck-and-the-conserva-liberal-flip-flop.html.

17. "Canada Announces Major Continued Support to Global Immunization," *Canadian International Development Agency (CIDA),* October 6, 2010, http://www.acdi-cida.gc.ca/acdi-cida/ACDI-CIDA.nsf/eng/NAT-10611287-L65.

18. "Merck Reports Double-Digit Earnings-Per-Share Growth for Second Quarter 2007," *Merck Newsroom,* July 23, 2007, http://www.merck.com/newsroom/news-release-archive/financial/2007_0723.html.

19. Sidney Tarrow, *Power in Movement: Social Movements and Contentious Politics* (Cambridge: Cambridge University Press, 2008).

20. Theodore Lowi, *The End of Liberalism* (New York: W. W. Norton Company, 1969) and Dorothy M. Stetson, "Abortion Triads and Women's Rights in Russia, the United States, and France," in *Abortion Politics: Public Policy in Cross-Cultural Perspective,* eds. Marianne Githens and Dorothy M. Stetson (New York: Routledge, 1996), 97–118.

21. Emanuela Lombardo, Petra Meier, and Mieke Verloo, "Stretching and Bending Gender Equality: A Discursive Politics Approach," in *The Discursive Politics of Gender Equality: Stretching, Bending and Policymaking,* eds. Emanuela Lombardo, Petra Meier and Mieke Verloo (London: Routledge, 2009), 5.

22. Ibid., 4.

23. Jacob Hacker, "Policy Drift: The Hidden Politics of US Welfare State Retrenchment," in *Beyond Continuity: Institutional Change in Advanced Political Economies,* eds. Wolfgang Streeck and Kathleen Thelen (Oxford: Oxford University Press, 2005), 40–82.

24. Frank Baumgartner and Bryan Jones, *Agendas and Instability in American Politics* (Chicago, IL: University of Chicago Press, 1993); Frank Baumgartner and Bryan Jones, eds., *Policy Dynamics* (Chicago, IL: University of Chicago Press, 2002); and Walter Dean Burnham, *Critical Elections: And the Mainsprings of American Politics* (New York: W. W. Norton and Company, 1971).

25. Wolfgang Streeck and Kathleen Thelen, "Introduction," in Streeck and Thelen, *Beyond Continuity,* 26.

26. Eliav Barr, Barry Buckland, and Kathrin Jansen, "The Story of Gardasil," *innovation.org,* http://www.innovation.org/index.cfm/StoriesofInnovation/InnovatorStories/The_Story_of_Gardasil.

27. Padmanabhan et al., "Intellectual Property," 671–78.

28. Mark Blaxill, "A License to Kill? Part 1: How a Public-Private Partnership Made the Government Merck's Gardasil Partner," *Age of Autism*, August 16, 2011, http://www.ageofautism.com/2010/05/a-license-to-kill-part-1-how-a-publicprivate-partnership-made-the-government-mercks-gardasil-partner.html.

29. Ibid.

30. Padmanabhan et al., "Intellectual Property," 671–78.

31. "FDA Approval History for Gardasil," *Drugs.com*, http://www.drugs.com/history/gardasil.html.

32. "Important Milestones in the History of FDA-Approved Plan B," *Reproductive Health Technologies Project*, December 13, 2011, http://www.rhtp.org/contraception/emergency/documents/ImportantMilestonesintheHistoryofFDAApprovedPlanB-Online_003.pdf.

33. "FDA Approval History for Cervarix," *Drugs.com*, http://www.drugs.com/history/cervarix.html.

34. Brandel France de Bravo, Maushami DeSoto, and Krystle Seu, "HPV: Q & A," *Cancer Prevention and Treatment Fund*, April 2009, http://www.stopcancerfund.org/posts/214.

35. Emma Hitt, "ACIP Recommends HPV Vaccine for 11- to 12-Year-Old Boys," *Medscape Medical News*, October 25, 2011, http://affectus.webnode.pt/news/acip-recommends-hpv-vaccine-for-11-to-12-year-old-boys1/.

36. Ibid.

37. Alexandra Stewart, "Childhood Vaccine and School Entry Requirements: The Case of HPV Vaccine," *Public Health Reports* 123, no. 6 (November–December 2008): 801–3, http://www.ncbi.nlm.nih.gov/pmc/articles/PMC2556726/.

38. Angela Zimm and Justin Bloom, "Merck Promotes Cervical Cancer Shot by Publicizing Viral Cause," *Bloomberg News*, May 26, 2006, http://www.bloomberg.com/apps/news?pid=newsarchive&sid=amVj.y3Eynz8.

39. Ibid.

40. The 1996 act amended previous immigration statutes and included in Section 341 the requirement that those in the United States filing for visas or change of status after September 30, 1996 had to show proof of multiple vaccinations.

41. The figures for the abstinence-based education program are from "A Brief History: Abstinence-Only-Until-Marriage Programs," *No More Money*, 2008, http://www.nomoremoney.org/index.cfm?pageid=947 and the data on Gardasil come from Zimm and Blum, "Merck Promotes Cervical Cancer."

42. Judith Siers-Poisson, "Research, Develop, and Sell, Sell, Sell: Part 2 in a Series on the Politics and PR of Cervical Cancer," *PR Watch*, June 30, 2007, http://prwatch.org/node/6208/.

43. Ross Ramsey, Jay Root, and Jim Rutenberg, "Texas Lobbyist Mike Toomey Is Force behind Rick Perry," *The New York Times*, October 14, 2011, http://www.texastribune.org/texas-politics/2012-presidential-election/in-perrys-texas-the-man-behind-the-curtain/.

44. "Rick Perry—Gardasil," *The Political Guide*, September 26, 2011, http://www.thepoliticalguide.com/Profiles/Governor/Texas/Rick_Perry/Scandals/Gardasil/.

45. Ibid.

46. Ibid.

47. "State Policies in Brief: State Funding of Abortion under Medicaid," *Guttmacher Institute*, http://www.guttmacher.org/statecenter/spibs/spib_SFAM.pdf.

48. "Rick Perry—Gardasil," *The Political Guide*.

49. Dan Eggen, "Perry's Financial Ties to Merck Run Deep," *The Washington Post*, September 14, 2011, http://www.thefiscaltimes.com/Articles/2011/09/14/WP-Perrys-Finan cial-Ties-to-Merck-Run-Deep.aspx#page1.

50. Nicholas Confessore and Michael Luo, "Perry Mines Texas System to Raise Cash for Campaigns," *The New York Times*, August 20, 2011, A1, http://www.nytimes. com/2011/08/21/us/politics/21donate.html?pagewanted=all.

51. Ramsey, Root, and Rutenberg, "Texas Lobbyist Mike Toomey."

52. Ibid.

53. Siers-Poisson, "Research, Develop, and Sell, Sell, Sell."

54. Ibid.

55. "Our Mission," Step Up Women's Network, http://www.suwn.org/mission.aspx.

56. Siers-Poisson, "Research, Develop, and Sell, Sell, Sell" and Laura Mamo, Amber Nelson, and Aleia Clark, "Producing and Protecting Risky Girlhoods," in *Three Shots at Prevention: The HPV Vaccine and the Politics of Medicine's Simple Solutions*, eds. Keith Wailoo, Julie Livingston, Steven Epstein, and Robert Aronowitz (Baltimore, MD: Johns Hopkins University Press, 2010): 121–45.

57. Mamo, Nelson and Clark, "Producing and Protecting Risky Girlhoods," 134–35.

58. These comparisons were made from two organizations' websites, www.ncsl.org and www.womeningovernment.org.

59. Judith Siers-Poisson, "Women in Government, Merck's Trojan Horse: Part 3 in a Series on the Politics and PR of Cervical Cancer," *PR Watch*, July 10, 2007, http:// prwatch.org/node/6232/.

60. Ibid.

61. QIAGEN, www.qiagen.com.

62. Siers-Poisson, "Women in Government, Merck's Trojan Horse."

63. Ibid.

64. Ibid.

65. "Childcare and School Immunization Requirements 2005–2006," Centers for Disease Control (CDC), p. 38, http://www2a.cdc.gov/nip/schoolsurv/ImmunizationRequire ments05_06.pdf and see also Stewart, "Childhood Vaccine and School Entry Requirements."

66. "HPV Vaccine," *National Conference of State Legislatures (NCSL)*, http://www. ncsl.org/issues-research/health/hpv-vaccine-state-legislation-and-statutes.aspx.

67. Ibid.

68. "An Analysis by the National Vaccine Information Center of Gardasil & Menactra Adverse Event Reports to the Vaccine Adverse Events Reporting System (VAERS)," *National Vaccine Information Center (NVIC)*, February 2009, http://www.nvic. org/downloads/nvicgardasilvsmenactravaersreportfeb-2009u.aspx.

8

Conclusion: Why a Feminist Historical Institutionalist Lens Is Important

There are many types of institutionalist theories, scrutinized from a feminist lens, that have helped provide an understanding of the evolution of the Food and Drug Administration (FDA) from 1930 onward and its relationship to the world's most profitable system of pharmas. Some non-institutionalist studies have been helpful as well. This book was bookended by two strange case studies. The first concerning the Pill discussed pharma's reticence to get behind the first prescription medicine taken long term by healthy women. The last concerning Gardasil highlighted the oddities in the process surrounding FDA approval and Merck's marketing of the first anti-cancer vaccine. Some of the oddities in the Gardasil approvals and marketing pipeline included Merck's co-optation of a group claiming to represent women state legislators and anti-cancer groups formed by women. Another set of strange events was seen in the actions of purportedly social conservative Texas governor Rick Perry, willing to mandate Gardasil's usage, and Medicaid funding for it. In between, the two case studies of RU-486 (mifepristone) and the morning-after pill, first the combination pill Preven and then the levonorgestrel-only Plan B yielded evidence as to how women's interests fared during the second policy period on U.S. women's reproductive drug policymaking. It has been shown that social conservative and companies' financial interests can line up along the same oppositional side of an issue as long as it concerns a women's drug, including the RU-486 and Plan B case studies. With regard to RU-486, the Searle company did not wish to have the drug's importation as a relevant political issue, since it required misoprostol to be fully effective. Misoprostol was under patent to Searle as Cytotec for the U.S. distribution until 2000. Thus, a barrage of social conservative arguments against medical abortion in the United States and abroad served to obscure the heart of the matter, which was that Searle did not make enough from misoprostol to risk its profits on other drugs by being tied to the RU-486 controversy. While he was in office, the George H. W. Bush administration kept RU-486 out of the United States. While Bush had been Reagan's vice president, Donald Rumsfeld headed Searle (1977–1985).

For RU-486, the pro-choice and women's policy communities that had developed out of the old demographers' networks of the 1960s represented in the Princeton University Office of Population Research, the Mailman School of Public Health at Columbia University, and the Population Council, all worked to get either international or U.S. manufacturers for RU-486. No large U.S. pharma companies would get involved, citing the pro-life threats. Representatives from the demographers' community, the Population Council, the Feminist Majority Fund, particularly Eleanor Smeal, and Lawrence Lader of ARM worked to try to get the French-made pill imported or licensed to another company that would make the pill and then the pro-choice coalition could work out the distribution end of the equation. A Chinese manufacturer was found, Hoechst-Roussel licensed RU-486 to the Population Council, and a series of distribution companies were formed, including Danco for the United States and the company formed by Beverly Winikoff in 2003 in part for international distribution through the World Health Organization, Gynuity. Without the assistance of President Clinton and Health and Human Services (HHS) Secretary Donna Shalala in shepherding through negotiations, particularly where Hoechst was able to buy the highly profitable Marion Merrell Dow company, RU-486 probably would never have been made available on the U.S. market. Hoechst's reluctance to get involved in producing RU-486 for the U.S. market is highly ironic given that the company it bought (Marion Merrell Dow) was comprised of companies that had tried to foist thalidomide onto the U.S. market (Richardson Merrell) and that had made Agent Orange for the Vietnam War (Dow Chemical). Hoechst displayed no hesitation in buying the company.

A similar reluctance of large U.S. companies to get involved in producing Plan B was shown. Again, the irony of this stance leaps out at readers, since their stand was based on unproven profitability. This statement cannot be taken seriously, since Plan B (and Preven before it) comprise higher dosages of the same ingredients in birth-control pills. Each company making birth-control pills in the United States knows how hugely profitable that market has been. Once again, the women's pro-choice and demographers' communities swung into action, including Dr. James Trussell, director of the Princeton University Office for Population Research, and Sharon Camp, former vice president of Population Action International. She then became president of the Women's Capital Corporation, formed to distribute Plan B in the United States. Dr. Trussell's role was one of helping to construct a medically-based discourse promoting first Preven and then Plan B. In numerous articles co-authored with members of the Population Council and the Kaiser Foundation, the case has been made for emergency contraception as being far more effective and less costly to health systems than unwanted pregnancies and abortion.[1] Dr. Camp has also functioned as coordinator and convener of the International Consortium for Emergency Contraception.[2] Plan B is owned by Teva Pharmaceuticals.

The benefits of conducting a feminist institutionalist study of the evolution of the U.S. pharma system on women's reproductive drugs enable the pinpointing of continuities and more abrupt ruptures according to the punctuated equilibrium model. Continuities were seen in the rhetoric and tactics of the Comstockian social conservatives of the late 19th and early 20th centuries and the social conservatives of a hundred years later. Both sets of actors claimed that sex should occur only in marriage and that following that model, birth control and abortion are not necessary. They also used the U.S. Customs Service and trade legislation to keep many U.S. women from accessing knowledge of birth control and samples of it.

Another continuity in the development of the U.S. pharma policy system over time is that purported concerns for a profit motive can work in virtually any context as an excuse by pharma companies not to provide women's reproductive drugs. For example, Searle would not fund research into the pill in the 1950s and large U.S. pharma companies were adverse to being involved with RU-486 and Plan B. On the other hand, when women received quick access to one drug, such as Gardasil, it was not from a pro-feminist stance but rather Merck's financial need to get a blockbuster drug approved. In the first policy system in the 1960s, women received access to publicly-funded contraception, but the United States was the secondary target of global demographers. An important related continuity is that the existence of well-heeled foundations, including those of McCormick, Rockefeller, PATH, Pathfinder, Buffett, Soros, the Population Council and the International Planned Parenthood Federation, has enabled the work of contraceptive and medical abortion development to continue during the decades when the U.S. government and pharma are engaged in an iteration of their codependent refusal to support these items. In other words, women's needs are more often than not held hostage to games that are played with their bodies and lives in one part of the policy system or another.

The early reputational struggles of the FDA from the 1930s until the 1960s enabled it to gain powers to keep drugs off the market in the interests of safety and efficacy. While the FDA has used these concepts well at times, particularly on the thalidomide issue, there are other times, especially during the second policy period, when it has not used these powers wisely. These were the import alert against RU-486 and the stretching out of the process for Plan B's approval, ultimately over-the-counter (OTC) for those 18 and older (later lowered to 17) from 1998 to 2006.

The historical institutionalist concepts of layering and conversion have been particularly helpful to this study, especially because layering shows continuity in institutions over time while conversion shows more sudden change, akin to Baumgartner and Jones's policy punctuations.[3] Conversion is particularly apt for the Republican-led second policy period, in which the FDA, HHS, and Title V of the Social Security Act and Title X of the Public Health Services Act were all turned toward conservative purposes. Also, drift was consciously made part of the process when fewer women had access to publicly-paid services than before the second policy period. Layering of both liberalizing and regressive policies onto the women's drug policy system has been discussed. Liberalizing trends certainly were shown when Margaret Sanger and Katherine McCormick funded the development of the Pill and it was approved by the FDA. Conservative layering has been shown in that President Obama's administration has kept a faith-based office in the White House and funding in the budget for abstinence-based policies (with Congress's help). Similarly, the issue of not wanting to campaign on making Plan B completely OTC for all ages was shared by President Clinton, his successor, George W. Bush in 2000 and 2004, and most recently, President Obama when HHS secretary Kathleen Sebelius turned down the idea.

There have been high-profile defenses of women's rights to contraception and abortion by courageous women in Congress, in many instances covered in the case studies. Ironically, women's access to publicly-funded contraception and abortion occurred during the first policy period when women were in single-digit percentages in Congress. Women only attained double-digit representation in 1992, well after the damage had been wrought in the Reagan and George H. W. Bush years, and just ahead of the conservative Gingrich Congress. Since 1992, pro-choice women in Congress and in the Executive branch have fought for women's continued access to contraception and abortion. A high-profile example of a woman's action at HHS included the resignation of Dr. Susan Wood, Assistant Commissioner for Public Health, in 2005 over the politicization of the FDA's approvals process on Plan B.

In addition to a feminist interpretation of historical institutionalist, punctuated equilibrium, and the political process models, other theories were helpful to explaining the policy puzzle that is the U.S. pharma system regarding women. It is true that in normal times, Lowi's iron triangle prevails, in which women are generally shut out of decision-making on reproductive drugs.[4] The development of the policy triad theory by Stetson and its use here to explain reproductive politics showed two windows of opportunity for women, both under the Clinton administration.[5] The windows were seized on both by highly experienced actors in the reproductive policy field, including demographic community organizations from the 1960s, and Lawrence Lader, follower of Margaret Sanger. Second-wave feminist organizations, such as the National Organization for Women, the Feminist Majority Foundation, NARAL, and the Center for Reproductive Rights, also helped push for RU-486 and Plan B OTC.

With respect to feminist discursive institutionalism as framed by Lombardo et al., it was possible to trace examples for all four of their models.[6] The Pill was the first form of chemical contraception for women and freed women from having to make contraceptive provisions at the time of sexual intercourse. It is therefore easy to describe the policy discourse surrounding its development as an example of equality stretching.[7] At the same time, opponents of contraception, including conservative religions, framed the Pill's development as fixing women's equality in a specific notion of women's autonomy.[8] Conservatives from the 1960s onward, particularly after the U.S. Supreme Court's 1973 *Roe v. Wade* decision, alluded to sexually liberated women as the chief reason for a purported societal downfall in the United States. It is also hypothesized here that the agreement forged by HHS Secretary Donna Shalala, President Bill Clinton, and representatives of the Population Council and the Hoechst-Roussel company to shift the RU-486 patent to the Population Council was an example of stretching women's equality. The evidence for this hypothesis is shown in that RU-486 was the first dedicated medical abortion regime for women, freeing them from having to go to an abortion clinic to encounter harassment and protests.

In terms of Lombardo et al.'s discursive institutionalist framework and the relevance to historical institutionalist models, it was also theorized here that the processes of layering RU-486 and Plan B onto the existing reproductive rights policy regime were examples of shrinking. Ironically, while making RU-486 available in the United States was a stretching of women's equality, with respect to women's reproductive rights, the advent of both RU-486 and Plan B could also be seen as shrinking women's equality to these specific aspects of reproductive provision. Finally, the layering of Gardasil onto the existing system was identified as an example of bending according to Lombardo et al.[9] In this example, Merck persuaded many women's groups, including anti-cancer groups such as the Cancer Research and Prevention Fund and the Step Up Women's Network, the Women in Government, and state legislators' associations to work with it in getting FDA approval for Gardasil and state mandating of vaccinations. While many women were convinced by Merck that the Gardasil vaccine was a crucial ingredient in preventing cervical cancer in the United States, evidence has since proven otherwise both to its efficacy and the fact it is much more needed globally. The public discourse to sell Gardasil was a prime example of discursive bending, in which women's interests and equality were not at the center.

This book has shown that the United States provides the most complicated framework for women's reproductive rights advocates, for many reasons. The first, highlighted in this study is the for-profit nature of the pharma system, its autonomy in decision-making, and protection from foreign competition. Daniel Carpenter has noted the irony of increasing the FDA's regulatory powers and companies' responsibility to keep in close contact with the FDA under legislative amendments to the 1938 Food Drug and Cosmetic Act. The result has been that "US regulation has converted the pharmaceutical firm from a 'producer' to a 'sponsor.'"[10] The second problematic aspect of the U.S. system, concerning health insurance and health service provision, is its decentralized nature. In 2003, Bovbjerg et al. termed the U.S. system at the top of the list of decentralization of health-care provision in federated systems.[11] The decentralization of the U.S. health-care decision-making system, plus the fact that the bulk of health-care insurance is privately-provided are intensely problematic for creating a nationally-consistent framework for women's reproductive drugs provision. In short, states and insurance companies can do almost whatever they want, within constitutional limits. Additionally, the passage of conscience-clause legislation in the majority of states means that women can still be refused any of the four drugs studied here. In terms of specific examples, women in 9 U.S. states live under a collaborative practice framework in which the nationally-mandated requirement of prescription status under age 17 for Plan B access is irrelevant. In the other 41 states, that restriction is quite relevant. Similarly, since the passage of the federal Hyde Amendment in 1976 and the passage of similar legislation at the state levels, states can refuse to pay for abortions. This includes medical abortion, RU-486. Since according to the Guttmacher Institute, 4 out of every 10 women of reproductive age live under the federally-defined poverty level, the Hyde framework is as problematic as its intention.

The bottom line for the U.S. system of political decision-making and reproductive drugs provision is that political will demonstrated at the federal level, such as under the Clinton administration's FDA approval of Plan B by prescription and RU-486, is necessary but not sufficient to stretch the notion of gender equality in reproductive rights to reach all women. States and private entities have an inordinate amount of power in reproductive services delivery in the United States, and national political will usually cannot force these groups to undertake a particular endeavor. Two potential improvements to the U.S. pharma policymaking system would include the following. Following the U.S. Supreme Court's June 28, 2012, decision in *National Federation of Independent Business et al. vs. Sebelius, Secretary of Health and Human Services*, the mandate for states to provide affordable insurance and for citizens to avail themselves of it remains. On the other hand, numerous lawsuits about the scope of the coverage remain, many of them brought by the Catholic church about providing birth control benefits to employees. Without consistent coverage for contraception at the very least, including Plan B, women will simply not have control over their reproductive lives. The United States will continue to have the highest unplanned pregnancy and abortion rates in the industrialized world. The second necessary but not sufficient improvement requires more women at the senior levels of the pharma iron triangle in the United States, including at least 30 percent in Congress, not likely to happen soon, and feminist women in the Oval Office.

NOTES

1. "James Trussell," *Princeton University*, http://www.princeton.edu/~trussell/.

2. "Sharon L. Camp, President and CEO," *Guttmacher Institute*, http://www.guttm acher.org/media/experts/camp.html.

3. Wolfgang Streeck and Kathleen Thelen, "Introduction: Institutional Change in Advanced Political Economies," and Jacob Hacker, "Policy Drift: The Hidden Politics of US Welfare State Retrenchment," in *Beyond Continuity: Institutional Change in Advanced Political Economies*, eds. Wolfgang Streeck and Kathleen Thelen (Oxford: Oxford University Press, 2005), 1–39 and 40–82; Frank Baumgartner and Bryan Jones, *Agendas and Instability in American Politics* (Chicago, IL: University of Chicago Press, 1993); and Frank Baumgartner and Bryan Jones, eds., *Policy Dynamics* (Chicago, IL: University of Chicago Press, 2002).

4. Theodore Lowi, *The End of Liberalism* (New York: Norton, 1969).

5. Dorothy M. Stetson, "Abortion Triads and Women's Rights in Russia, the United States, and France," in *Abortion Politics: Public Policy in Cross-Cultural Perspective*, eds. Marianne M. Githens and Dorothy M. Stetson (New York: Routledge, 1996), 97–118.

6. Emanuela Lombardo, Petra Meier, and Mieke Verloo, "Stretching and Bending Gender Equality: A Discursive Approach," in *The Discursive Politics of Gender Equality: Stretching, Bending and Policymaking*, eds. Emanuela Lombardo, Petra Meier and Mieke Verloo (London: Routledge, 2009), 1–18.

7. Ibid., 5.

8. Ibid., 3.

9. Ibid., 5–6.

10. Daniel Carpenter, *Reputation and Power: Organizational Image and Pharmaceutical Regulation at the FDA* (Princeton, NJ: Princeton University Press, 2010), 637.

11. Randall R. Bovbjerg, Joshua M. Wiener, and Michael Houseman, "State and Federal Roles in Healthcare: Rationales for Allocating Responsibilities," in *Federalism and Health Policy,* eds. John Holahan, Alan Weil, and Joshua M. Wiener (Washington, DC: Urban Institute, July 2003), 30.

Selected Bibliography

Ahearn, Raymond. *US Trade Policy and Changing Foreign and Domestic Priorities: A Historical Overview*. CRS Report RS21657. Washington, DC: Congressional Research Service, November 3, 2003.

Angell, Marcia. *The Truth about the Drug Companies: How They Deceive Us and What to Do about It*. New York: Random House, 2005.

Annas, George J. and Sherman Elias. "Thalidomide and the *Titanic*: Reconstructing the Technology Tragedies of the Twentieth Century." *American Journal of Public Health* 89, no. 1 (January 1999): 98–101.

Bachrach, Peter and Morton S. Baratz. "Two Faces of Power." *American Political Science Review* 56, no. 4 (December 1962): 947–52.

Baer, Judith A. *Our Lives before the Law: Constructing a Feminist Jurisprudence*. Princeton, NJ: Princeton University Press, 1999.

Baumgartner, Frank and Bryan Jones, eds. *Agendas and Instability in American Politics*. Chicago, IL: University of Chicago Press, 1993.

Baumgartner, Frank and Bryan Jones, eds. *Policy Dynamics*. Chicago, IL: University of Chicago Press, 2002.

Beisel, Nicola. *Imperiled Innocents: Anthony Comstock and Family Reproduction in Victorian America*. Princeton, NJ: Princeton University Press, 1997.

Beyeler, Michelle and Claire Annesley. "Gendering the Institutional Reform of the Welfare State: Germany, the United Kingdom, and Switzerland." In *Gender, Politics and*

Institutions: Towards a Feminist Institutionalism, edited by Mona Lena Krook and Fiona Mackay, 79–94. New York: Palgrave Macmillan, 2011.

Bovbjerg, Randall R., Joshua M. Wiener, and Michael Houseman. "State and Federal Roles in Healthcare: Rationales for Allocating Responsibilities." In *Federalism and Health Policy*, edited by John Holahan, Alan Weil, and Joshua M. Wiener, 25–57. Washington, DC: Urban Institute, 2003.

Burnham, Walter Dean. *Critical Elections: And the Mainsprings of American Politics*. New York: W. W. Norton and Company, 1971.

Carpenter, Daniel. *The Forging of Bureaucratic Autonomy: Reputation, Networks and Policy Innovation in Executive Agencies, 1862–1928*. Princeton, NJ: Princeton University Press, 2001.

Carpenter, Daniel. *Reputation and Power: Organizational Image and Pharmaceutical Regulation at the FDA*. Princeton, NJ: Princeton University Press, 2010.

Ceccoli, Stephen. *Pill Politics: Drugs and the FDA*. Boulder, CO: Lynne Rienner, 2003.

Charnovitz, Steve. "The Moral Exception in Trade Policy." 38 *Virginia Journal of International Law* 689 (Summer 1998): 1–49.

Chicoine, Denise. "RU-486 in the US and Great Britain: A Case Study in Gender Bias." *Boston College International and Comparative Law Review* 16, no. 1 (December 1993): 81–113.

Coleman, Clare and Kirtly Parker Jones. "Title X: A Proud Past, an Uncertain Future." *Contraception* 84, no. 3 (2011): 209–11.

Confessore, Nicholas and Michael Luo. "Perry Mines Texas System to Raise Cash for Campaigns." *New York Times*, August 20, 2011, A1.

Critchlow, Donald. *Intended Consequences: Birth Control, Abortion and the Federal Government in Modern America*. New York: Oxford University, 2001.

Crouse, Lynda. "*Benten v. Kessler:* The Time for Uniformity in the Application of Section 553 of the Administrative Procedure Act Has Come." *The American University Administrative Law Journal* 7, no. 2 (Summer 1993): 344–71.

Doan, Alesha E. and Jean Calterone Williams. *The Politics of Virginity: Abstinence in Sex Education*. Westport, CT: Praeger, 2008.

Ellertson, Charlotte. "History and Efficacy of Emergency Contraception: Beyond Coca Cola." *Family Planning Perspectives* 28, no. 2 (March–April 1996): 44–48.

Ellison, Sara Fisher and Wallace P. Mullin. "Gradual Incorporation of Information: Pharmaceutical Stocks and the Evolution of President Clinton's Health Care Reform." *Journal of Law and Economics* XLIV, no. 1 (April 2001): 89–129.

Evans, Peter B., Dietrich Rueschmeyer, and Theda Skocpol, eds. *Bringing the State Back in*. Cambridge: Cambridge University Press, 1985.

Graham, Edward M. and David M. Marchick. *US National Security and Foreign Direct Investment*. Washington, DC: Institute for International Economics, 2006.

Greer, Scott L. and Bert Vanhercke. "The Hard Politics of Soft Law: The Case of Health." In *Health Systems Governance in Europe: The Role of European Union Law and Policy*, edited by Elias Mossialos et al., 186–230. Cambridge: Cambridge University Press, 2010.

Hacker, Jacob. "Policy Drift: The Hidden Politics of US Welfare State Retrenchment." In *Beyond Continuity: Institutional Change in Advanced Political Economies*, edited by

Wolfgang Streeck and Kathleen Thelen, 40–82. Oxford: Oxford University Press, 2005.

Haussman, Melissa. *Abortion Politics in North America*. Boulder, CO: Lynne Rienner, 2005.

Haussman, Melissa. "Caught in a Bind: The US Pro-Choice Movement and Federalism." In *Federalism, Feminism and Multilevel Governance*, edited by Melissa Haussman, Marian Sawer, and Jill Vickers, 111–26. Surrey: Ashgate, 2010.

Haussman, Melissa and David Biette. "Buy American or Buy Canadian? Public Procurement Politics and Policy under International Frameworks." In *How Ottawa Spends, 2010–2011: Recession, Realignment and the New Deficit Era*, edited by G. Bruce Doern and Christopher Stoney, 121–49. Montreal: McGill-Queen's University Press, 2010.

Haussman, Melissa and Pauline Rankin. "Framing the Harper Government: 'Gender-Neutral' Electoral Appeals while Being Gender-Negative in Caucus." In *How Ottawa Spends, 2009–2010: Economic Upheaval and Political Dysfunction*, edited by Allan M. Maslove, 241–62. Montreal: McGill-Queen's University Press, 2009.

Hawthorne, Fran. *Inside the FDA: The Business and Politics Behind the Drugs We Take and the Food We Eat*. Hoboken, NJ: John Wiley and Sons, 2005.

Hilts, Philip J. *Protecting America's Health: The FDA, Business, and One Hundred Years of Regulation*. Chapel Hill, NC: University of North Carolina Press, 2003.

Hollander, Ilyssa. "Viagra's Rise above Women's Health Issues: An Analysis of the Social and Political Influences on Drug Approvals in the US and Japan." *Social Sciences and Medicine* 62, no. 3 (2006): 683–93.

Jackson, Charles. *Food and Drug Legislation in the New Deal*. Princeton, NJ: Princeton University Press, 1970.

Johnson, Judith. *Abortion: Termination of Early Pregnancy with RU-486 (Mifepristone)*. CRS Report RL 30866. Washington, DC: Congressional Research Service, February 23, 2011.

Kingdon, John. *Agendas, Alternatives and Public Policies*, 2nd ed. London: Longman and Pearson, 1984.

Kort, Michele. "Denial by Delay." *Ms.* (Spring 2006): xvi, 1, 12.

Krook, Mona Lena and Fiona Mackay. "Introduction: Gender, Politics and Institutions." In *Gender, Politics and Institutions*, edited by Mona Lena Krook and Fiona Mackay, 1–20. New York: Palgrave Macmillan, 2011.

Lader, Lawrence. *A Private Matter: RU-486 and the Abortion Crisis*. Amherst, NY: Prometheus Books, 1995.

Lombardo, Emanuela, Petra Meier, and Mieke Verloo. "Stretching and Bending Gender Equality: A Discursive Politics Approach." In *The Discursive Politics of Gender Equality: Stretching, Bending and Policymaking*, edited by Emanuela Lombardo, Petra Meier, and Mieke Verloo, 1–18. Oxon: Routledge, 2009.

Lowi, Theodore J. *The End of Liberalism: Ideology, Policy, and the Crisis of Authority*. New York: Norton, 1969.

Mackay, Fiona. "Toward a Feminist Institutionalism?" In *Gender, Politics and Institutions*, edited by Mona Lena Krook and Fiona Mackay, 181–96. New York: Palgrave Macmillan, 2011.

Mamo, Amber Nelson and Aleia Clark. "Producing and Protecting Risky Girlhoods." In *Three Shots at Prevention: The HPV Vaccine and the Politics of Medicine's Simple Solutions*, edited by Keith Wailoo, Julie Livingston, Steven Epstein, and Robert Aronowitz, 121–45. Baltimore, MD: The Johns Hopkins University Press, 2010.

March, James G. and Johan P. Olsen. "The New Institutionalism: Organizational Factors in Political Life." *The American Political Science Review* 78, no. 2 (1984): 734–49.

Marks, Lara V. *Sexual Chemistry: A History of the Contraceptive Pill*. New Haven, CT: Yale University Press, 2010.

Mazur, Amy and Dorothy E. McBride. "Gendering New Institutionalism." In *The Politics of State Feminism: Innovation in Comparative Research*, edited by Dorothy E. McBride and Amy G. Mazur, 217–40. Philadelphia, PA: Temple University Press, 2010.

McAdam, Doug, John McCarthy, and Mayer Zald. *Comparative Perspectives on Social Movements: Political Opportunities, Mobilizing Structures and Cultural Framings*. Cambridge: Cambridge University Press, 1996.

Mundy, Alicia. "Political Lobbying Drove FDA Process." *Wall Street Journal*, March 6, 2009.

Phillips, Kevin. *The Emerging Republican Majority*. New York: Anchor, 1970.

Pierson, Paul. *Dismantling the Welfare State? Reagan, Thatcher, and the Politics of Retrenchment*. Cambridge: Cambridge University Press, 1994.

Ramsey, Ross, Jay Root, and Jim Rutenberg. "Texas Lobbyist Mike Toomey Is Force behind Rick Perry." *Texas Tribune*, October 14, 2011.

Reagan, Leslie J. *When Abortion Was a Crime: Women, Medicine and the Law in the US, 1867–1973*. Berkeley, CA: University of California Press, 1998.

Reed, James. *The Birth Control Movement and American Society: From Private Vice to Public Virtue*. Princeton, NJ: Princeton University Press, 1984.

Saletan, William. *Bearing Right: How Conservatives Won the Abortion War*. Berkeley, CA: University of California Press, 2004.

Schroedel, Jean Reith and Tanya Buhler Corbin. "Gender Relations and Institutional Conflict over Mifepristone." *Women & Politics* 24, no. 3 (2002): 35–60.

Sinclair, Barbara. *Unorthodox Lawmaking: New Legislative Processes in the U.S. Congress*, 3rd ed. Washington, DC: Congressional Quarterly, Inc., 2007.

Skowronek, Stephen. *Building a New American State: The Expansion of National Administrative Capacities, 1877–1920*. Cambridge: Cambridge University Press, 1982.

Stetson, Dorothy M. "Abortion Triads and Women's Rights in Russia, the United States, and France." In *Abortion Politics: Public Policy in Cross-Cultural Perspective*, edited by Marianne M. Githens and Dorothy M. Stetson, 97–118. New York: Routledge, 1996.

Stewart, Alexandra. "Childhood Vaccine and School Entry Requirements: The Case of HPV Vaccine." *Public Health Reports* 123, no. 6 (November–December 2008): 801–3.

Streeck, Wolfgang and Kathleen Thelen. "Introduction: Institutional Change in Advanced Political Economies." In *Beyond Continuity: Institutional Change in Advanced Political Economies*, edited by Wolfgang Streeck and Kathleen Thelen, 1–39. Oxford: Oxford University Press, 2005.

Sundquist, James L. *Dynamics of the Party System: The Growth and Realignment of Political Parties in the US*, revised ed. Washington, DC: Brookings, 1983.

Talaga, Tanya. "Lobbyists Boosted Vaccine Program." *Toronto Star,* August 16, 2007.

Tarrow, Sidney. *Power in Movement: Social Movements and Contentious Politics.* Cambridge: Cambridge University Press, 1998.

Thelen, Kathleen. "How Institutions Evolve: Insights from Comparative Historical Analysis." In *Comparative Analysis in the Social Sciences,* edited by James Mahoney and Dietrich Rueschemeyer, 208–40. Cambridge: Cambridge University Press, 2003.

Trussell, James, Charlotte Ellertson, and Felicia Stewart, "The Effectiveness of the Yuzpe Regimen of Emergency Contraception," *Family Planning Perspectives* 28, no. 2 (March–April 1996): 58–64, 97.

Watkins, Elizabeth Siegel. *On the Pill: A Social History of Oral Contraceptives, 1950–1970.* Baltimore, MD: The Johns Hopkins University Press, 1998.

Yuzpe, A. A. et al. "Post Coital Contraception: A Pilot Study." *Journal of Reproductive Medicine* 13, no. 2 (August 1974): 53–58.

Zimm, Angela and Justin Bloom. "Merck Promotes Cervical Cancer Shot by Publicizing Viral Cause." *Bloomberg News,* May 26, 2006.

Index

About the Author

MELISSA HAUSSMAN, PhD, is associate professor of political science at Carleton University, Ottawa, Canada. Her scholarship focuses on Canadian and U.S. political structures and behavior, particularly as they impact and include women. Haussman's published works include *Abortion Politics in North America; Gendering the State in the Age of Globalization: Women's Movements and State Feminism in Postindustrial Democracies*, co-edited with Birgit Sauer; and Federalism, *Feminism and Multilevel Governance*, co-edited with Marian Sawer and Jill Vickers.